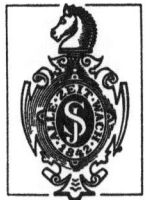

Klaus-Joachim Zülch

The Cerebral Infarct

Pathology, Pathogenesis, and
Computed Tomography

With 67 Figures
in 130 Separate Illustrations

Springer-Verlag
Berlin Heidelberg New York Tokyo

KLAUS-JOACHIM ZÜLCH, Prof. Dr. Dr. h.c.
Emeritus Director of the Max-Planck-Institute for Neurological Research
and of the Neurological Clinic of the City Hospital Köln-Merheim,
Ostmerheimerstraße 200, D-5000 Köln 91 (Merheim)

Enlarged from an invited paper presented at the World Congress of Neurology,
Kyoto, Japan, September 20–25, 1981

ISBN-13:978-3-642-70767-4   e-ISBN-13:978-3-642-70765-0
DOI: 10.1007/978-3-642-70765-0

Dedicated to
M. L.

Preface

The aim of this book is to expand the clinical information given by computed tomograms (CTs) of cerebral infarcts. Anatomical sections are displayed parallel to the CT correlate in the hope that the interpretation of pathogenesis will provide valuable clinical data at a time when the number of angiographies performed in cerebrovascular cases has diminished rapidly.

For better understanding of pathogenesis our concepts concerning the process of infarction have been summarized on the basis of schematic drawings.

Köln   K.-J. ZÜLCH

Acknowledgments

I am most grateful to Professor Hoeffken for permission to use computed tomograms from his institution, to Herr Göldner and Frau Mühlhöver for their technical assistance, and to Frau Göldner for help during the editorial work. My particular thanks go to my friend Professor W.S. Fields, Houston, who undertook the great burden of styling the English text.

My gratitude is expressed to Dr. Dr. h.c. mult. Heinz Götze and Springer-Verlag for the excellent layout and quality of this book.

The project was supported by a grant from Frau Andrea Möller, Hamburg.

Contents

I Cerebral Infarcts and Computed Tomograms

1 Introduction

Comparison of the morphology of cerebral infarcts observed in computed tomograms (CTs) with the anatomical specimens is important if the maximum information regarding pathogenesis is to be obtained from this non invasive diagnostic method. Such information should be helpful to the clinician.

The importance of such a comparison is demonstrated by the following:

1. The majority of radiologists or clinicians who are familiar with CTs of infarcts do not have the opportunity to study the postmortem appearance of brain infarcts and to compare them thoroughly with the radiological findings.
2. Many physicians are unaware of the highly developed and hemodynamically structured pathogenetic concept of infarction which exists today.
3. The classification of ischemic lesions, which includes
   a) TIA (transient ischemic attack)
   b) RIND (reversible ischemic neurologic deficit)
   c) Progressing stroke
   d) Completed stroke
   is derived from extent and duration, without consideration of pathogenesis. This classification, however, gives incomplete information regarding the lesion and its pathogenesis.
4. The clinician is extremely interested in having pathogenetic information in a case of stroke:
   a) Type of stroke (i.e., hemorrhage, infarction, embolism)
   b) Type of infarct (vascular occlusion, hemodynamic insufficiency, etc.)
   c) Exact location
   d) Role played by collateral circulation through anastomoses.

In the past many of these questions were answered by comparative study of "four-vessel angiography" and technetium (Tc) scintigraphy. Computed tomography provides much of the information, but without giving any representation of the circulation.

5. Although it is hoped that digital subtraction angiography will eventually provide sufficient information regarding the circulation, one should attempt to obtain maximum information from the CT scan.

Highly specialized angiography and Tc scintigraphy have aided in the development of current concepts of the pathogenesis of the various types of cerebral infarcts. It may be possible to determine which vessel is compromised and also the role of collateral circulation by analysis of the type of lesion seen on the CT scan. It is this possibility which has stimulated us to study the typical infarcts seen in a neurologic clinic and correlate them with a series of specimens obtained a decade earlier while we were investigating the pathogenesis of cerebral infarction (ZÜLCH and GESSAGA 1972). These pathological specimens were collected at a time during which a specific therapy for infarction was not being used at our institution. Although most of these cases are "virgin," they differ very little from the specimens we now obtain after attempts to treat infarction specifically.

This chapter will provide an introduction to our concepts of the pathogenesis of infarction, developed on the basis of experience both in the autopsy room and in the intensive care unit (see the correlated study in ZÜLCH 1981). The aim of the discussion, however, will be to demonstrate the increased amount of information which can be acquired from a correlated study of the CT and the pathomorphological pattern of infarction.

There are two ways of creating such a correlated study:

1. Classification of infarct patterns according to the location and type of the defect, i.e., occlusion of major arteries and branches, defects along border zones, lacunar infarction, etc., as attempted by VALK (1980)
2. Classification of infarcts by modern concepts of pathogenesis, making possible a stereotyped explanation for the tendency of common types of infarcts. This includes the designation of:
   a) The major irrigating vessel
   b) The type of lesion involving the vasculature
   c) The exact location of the resulting process
   d) The pattern of preexisting anastomoses and the resulting collateral systems
   e) The general hemodynamic and cardiovascular situation at the moment of the insult, including factors such as hypertensive crisis, hypotensive crisis, microcirculatory changes, alteration in viscosity of the blood, such as sludging and erythrocytosis, and the possibility of a microembolic lesion.

To make meaningful comparison of the CT scan and the tissue specimen, it is necessary to know the exact distribution of individual arteries. This vascular anatomy is well demonstrated in the atlases of SALAMON (1971) and SALAMON and HUANG (1976), or PERNKOPF (1957, 1960) and LANG (1981).

We want to emphasize our own experience, which refutes the common claim that only stenotic lesions of at least 75%–85% result in cerebrovascular insufficiency in the territory of supply beyond the stenosis. During hypotensive crisis, for example, lesions of 30%–50% can be of sufficient magnitude to provoke circulatory insufficiency. Moreover, it must be considered that retrograde flow may be hampered by preexisting anastomotic pathways which form a "physiological stenosis," decreasing the availability of collateral circulation when the primary vessel is blocked. Hypoxia is also able to precipitate infarction in an only slightly compromised vessel secondary to an additive decrease in oxygen delivery, as are metabolic changes.

In summary, any new information related to the pathogenesis of cerebral infarction or cerebrovascular insufficiency not only provides a step forward in academic knowledge, but also influences the nature and duration of any treatment program.

2 Incidence of Cerebral Infarcts in a Series of Unselected Computed Cranial Tomograms

This report is based on a review of approximately 12000 cranial CTs, of which around 9% showed infarcts. These included mainly cases seen on the neurological ward of the Merheim City Hospital during my directorship and that of my successor, Prof. W.D. Heiss, to whom I am grateful for permission to use some of the later cases in this discussion. The majority of the CT scans, which were performed on third- and fourth-generation scanners (General Electrics, CT 9800), were of outpatients who were referred by hospitals, general practitioners, and neurologists. This explains how serial sections and repeat CTs, desirable to follow the course of the lesion, were possible only in some cases.

3 Concept of Cerebral Infarction

For a better understanding of the pathogenesis of infarction, the laws relating the site of infarct to the involvement of the irrigating vessels must be discussed, starting with the classical concept put forth by COHNHEIM (1882). This concept assumes that blocking of cerebral end-arteries leads to infarction of the complete territory of supply (Fig. 1). The correlation

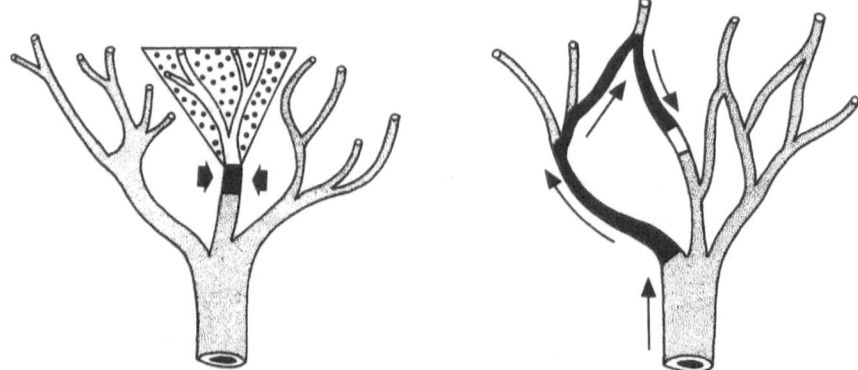

Fig. 1. **Left** Infarction by occlusion of an end-artery according to the concept of Cohnheim. **Right** Sequelae of this occlusion are prevented by anastomoses and a retrograde collateral supply

between occlusion of a cerebral artery and the occurrence and extent of infarction is now known to be far more complicated.

The blood supply to the brain is much more complex because of the extensive pattern of extra- and intracranial anastomoses, which provide collateral circulation between the four principal brain arteries in case of emergency (Figs. 1 and 9).

The principal anastomoses of the cerebral circulation which connect the four arteries extra- and intracranially are (see Figs. 2 and 3):

1. Between the two common carotid arteries
2. Between the external carotid artery and the vertebral artery
3. Between the external carotid artery and the intracranial circulation through anastomoses with the ophthalmic artery
4. Through the intracranial system of the circle of Willis at the base of the brain
5. Across the "meningeal anastomoses" of Heubner (HEUBNER 1872, 1874; VAN DER EECKEN and ADAMS 1953), which form a reticulum over the surface of the brain (Fig. 9)
6. Through the arterial ring anastomoses of SCHMIDT (1955, Fig. 3), the small annular arterial connections within the arachnoid which are known to play a role particularly in the thromboangiitis obliterans of Winiwarter-Buerger (Fig. 60). During typical arterial infarctions these, much like the capillary anastomoses of PFEIFER (1930, 1931), are practically without significance.

These interconnections, which provide the basis for collateral circulation, and their significance in relation to patterns of infarction will be discussed in detail. It is important, however, to mention that Cohnheim's theory of

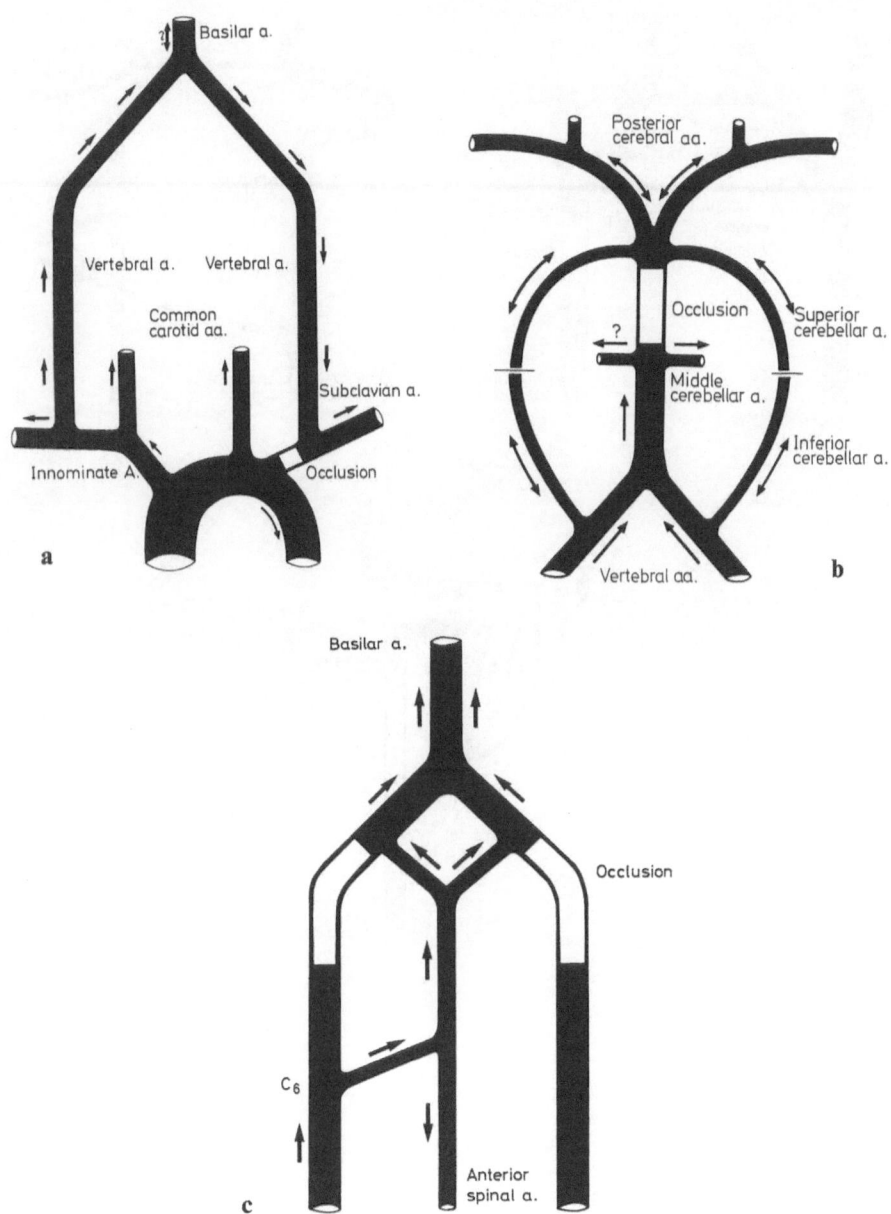

Fig. 2. a Confluence of the two vertebral arteries may provide a very long anastomotic source of supply in the case of occlusion of one subclavian artery. This may
even be temporarily detrimental to the basilar artery circulation (so-called subclavian
steal). **b** With occlusion of the basilar artery anastomoses between the posterior
inferior and superior cerebellar arteries may become operative. **c** With occlusion
of both vertebrals the anterior spinal artery can be used as a detour around the
obstruction

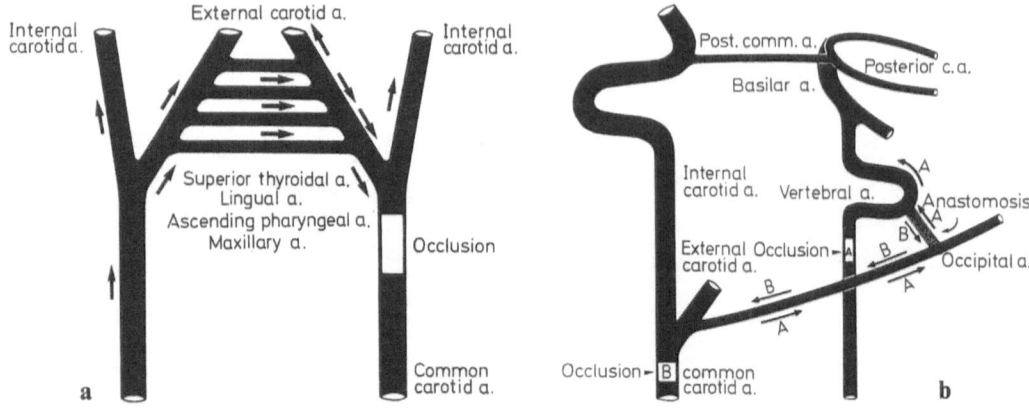

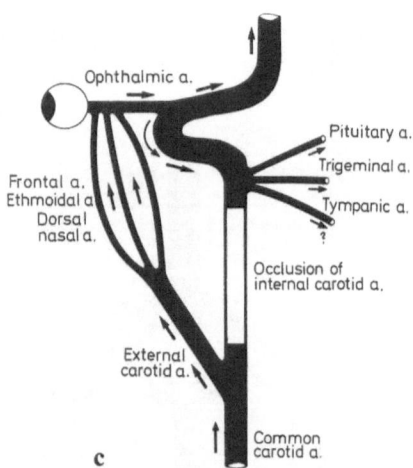

Fig. 3a–c. Schematic diagram of main anastomoses between the "four vessels" extra-
and intracranially. **a** Anastomoses between the two external carotid arteries through
numerous transverse branches in the neck. **b** The vertebral and the carotid systems
are connected by the greater occipital arterial channel which can work in either
direction following occlusion (*A* or *B*). **c** In a case of occlusion of the internal
carotid artery, anastomoses between the external and distal internal carotid artery
form a detour around the occlusion via the ophthalmic artery. The main communica-
tions are through the frontal, ethmoidal, or dorsal nasal arteries

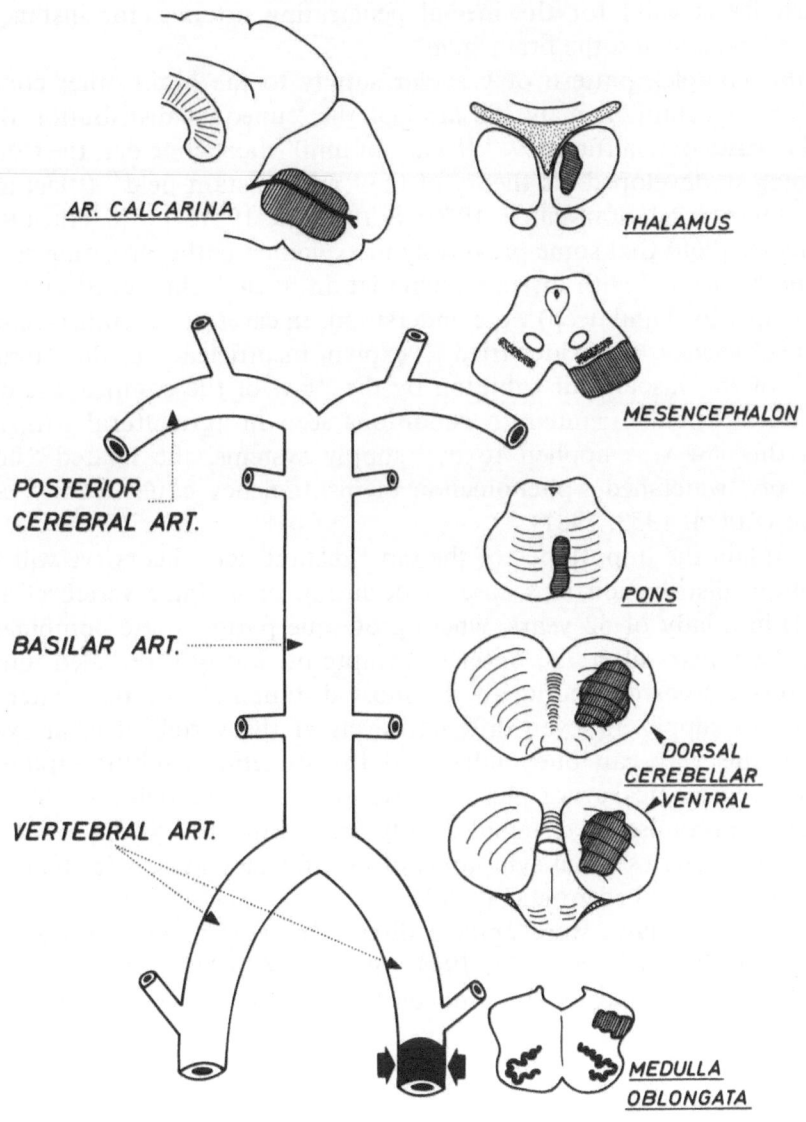

Fig. 4. Schematic drawing to show seven different levels of infarction in a case of occlusion of one vertebral artery. Defects of irrigation may involve either the total system or the center of the supply areas

end-arteries is valid for the medial penetrating arteries, for instance, of the basal ganglia and the brain stem.

In this complex pattern of vascular supply to the brain other concepts are also important, namely the laws of the "unequal distribution of the blood in cases of insufficiency." It was not until Max Schneider, the Cologne physiologist, developed his theory of the "most distant field" ("last meadow") (OPITZ and SCHNEIDER 1950; SCHNEIDER 1951, 1952; HIRSCH and SCHNEIDER 1968) that some previously unexplained pathophysiological phenomena associated with disrupted circulation in the spinal cord and in the brain (superficial and deep) were understood. In cases of generalized circulatory insufficiency, Schneider tried to explain insufficiency in the "terminal zones" of the vascular distribution by the "law of the compromise of the most distant field" (similar to conditions seen in agricultural irrigation). When this law was applied to two supply systems, the related "border zone" or "watershed" phenomenon of insufficiency could readily be explained (ZÜLCH 1953, 1981).

To explain the importance of the most distant field theory we will show the infarct distribution in a case of occlusion of a single vertebral artery (Fig. 4) in a lady of 52 years, where grotesque patterns and combinations arose. Two years after the onset of symptoms, autopsy revealed multiple small infarcts corresponding to the most distant field or the center of a territory of supply at seven different levels of the vertebrobasilar system. Only in this way can one understand the sometimes multisymptomatic, complex neurological syndrome of "vertebrobasilar insufficiency." This pattern of compromise in terminal supply areas can also be applied to two neighboring arteries when symptoms of insufficiency appear in the borderline zone or watershed zone (Fig. 5d).

These general laws were applied directly to study the pathogenesis of cerebral infarcts (ZÜLCH 1953, 1954, 1961, 1968, 1979, 1981) in order to explain hemodynamically this frequently unsystematic process (for details see ZÜLCH 1981).

3.1 General Semiology of Infarction

The main general patterns of infarction can be subdivided and explained in the following way (the processes and defects leading to the lesions will be described later).

1. On the *surface* of the brain, usually following general intracranial vascular insufficiency, superficial, semicircular infarcts can arise at the border of the territory of the middle cerebral artery. These infarcts involve the watershed areas between the middle cerebral artery on one side and the posterior and anterior cerebral arteries on the other (Fig. 5d). They can

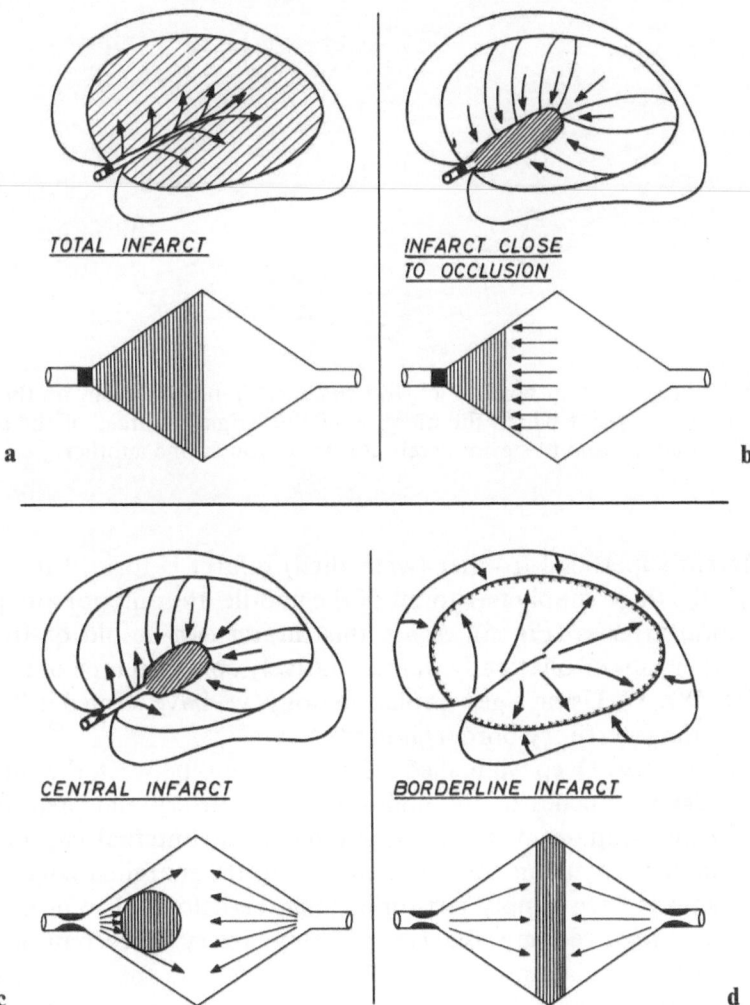

Fig. 5a–d. Various types and sizes of infarcts in different hemodynamic patterns.
a Total infarct due to defective collateral supply. **b** Peripheral zones supplied by
meningeal anastomoses of the neighborhood. **c** When stenosis rather than occlusion
is present, the infarcted area may be shifted into the center of the supply area.
In this case, the proximal parts are still directly supplied. **d** In the watershed (border
zone areas) of the three main arteries, cerebrovascular insufficiency may lead to
scars or infarcts

be fresh and are usually hemorrhagic, but can also present as old, deeply
scarred zones. They may also be seen in thromboangiitis obliterans of
Winiwarter-Buerger as granular atrophy (Fig. 59a) (LINDENBERG and
SPATZ 1940).

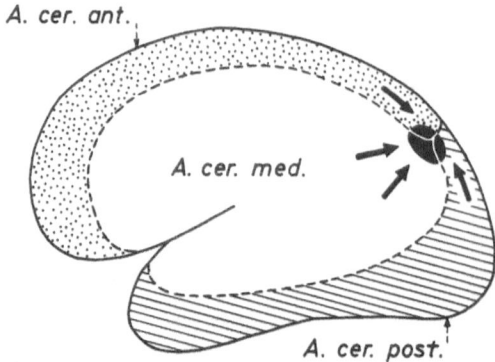

Fig. 6. The "three-territory border" (*"Dreiländereck"*) infarcts occur on the surface of the brain at the point where the margins of the irrigating areas of the anterior, middle, and posterior cerebral arteries touch one another

2. A different superficial frontier (watershed) infarct is formed in the zone between the three supply territories of the middle, the anterior and posterior cerebral arteries (Fig. 6). Again this infarct can be old or fresh and occur either uni- or bilaterally. It is a relatively common type of infarction (see Fig. 58a, b). Using a geographic analogy, we have termed it *"Dreiländereck"* (three-territory border) infarct.

3. *Deep Infarctions.* Deep watershed infarcts develop between the superficial and the deep branches of the middle cerebral artery and present themselves in the caudate nucleus, the putamen, and internal capsule. They follow the hemodynamic law of endangering the marginal zones (watersheds) between two supply territories (Fig. 12 below). The deep arteries most often involved are the central long artery (recurrent artery of Heubner), the medial and lateral striate arteries, and the anterior choroidal artery. In this pattern the superficial supply comes from the cortical branches of the middle cerebral artery (see Figs. 11 and 12). The borderline is near the putamen and the head of the caudate nucleus.

4. If the main stem of the middle cerebral artery is occluded the complete supply area can be infarcted, provided the general hemodynamic situation is poor and the anastomoses from the neighboring (anterior and posterior) cerebral arteries are not functioning. If, however, there is at least a partial supply through anastomoses, then only the proximal part of the supply area located near the stump (Fig. 5b) will be infarcted.

5. Infarction in the center of a supply area may occur if the stump is only stenosed (Fig. 5c). The proximal part of the supply area can be irrigated in the normal way, while the more distal parts receive an insufficient supply. However, the terminal zones of the supply area bordering on the irrigating area of the neighboring main arteries will obtain a sufficient

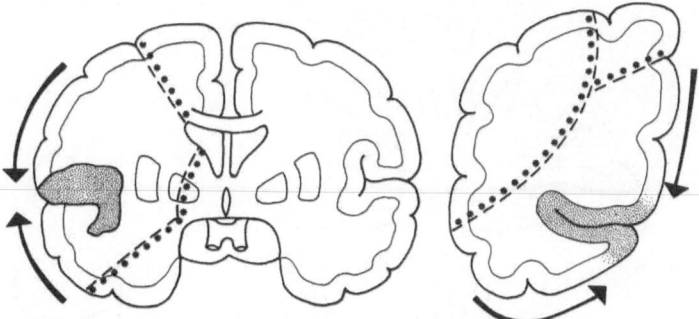

Fig. 7. Infarcts in the center of a supply area of the middle cerebral artery area involving frontal operculum and upper part of insula. In the posterior cerebral artery territory, the calcarine area is compromised. The Broca and calcarina centers are particularly compromised in special hemodynamic conditions

supply through the collateral systems. The actual area of insufficiency under these conditions will be located directly in the center of the original distribution (Fig. 5c). This is particularly well known in the territories of the middle and posterior cerebral arteries (Fig. 7).

Appreciation of these partial, centrally located infarcts is important for the interpretation of neurological symptomatology which will vary in relation to the collateral supply from the neighboring arteries. The infarcted area (Fig. 5a) may shrink, depending on the site of occlusion (Fig. 65) and amount of anastomotic supply. It may shrink concentrically when collateral flow is inadequate (Fig. 10). For example, in the distribution of the middle cerebral artery this center infarct will be located near the frontal, parietal and temporal operculum and in parts of the insula. On the left it may involve Broca's speech area (Fig. 7; ZÜLCH 1961). Its CT pattern has only recently been discovered (Fig. 20a, b).

In the territory of the posterior cerebral artery, the primary visual center of the calcarine cortex may be involved by this type of infarct in the center (ZÜLCH 1961; KLEIHUES and HIZAWA 1966; ZÜLCH and KLEIHUES 1967).

Since the clinical syndromes related to infarction of the center territory of a cerebral artery are not uncommon, it is important for the neurologist to recognize that they are usually present as a single symptom such as, possibly, a slight facial paresis, expressive/motor aphasia (left middle cerebral artery), or a (partial?) hemianopic defect (posterior cerebral artery).

6. Very curious but typical microinfarcts of the lacunar type are observed in the most distant field of a supply area. They may present as twin phenomena, (a) in the white matter of the semioval center, and/or (b) at the periphery of the putamen or caudate nucleus (Fig. 8). These typically localized lacunae can also be observed bilaterally. Our interpretation

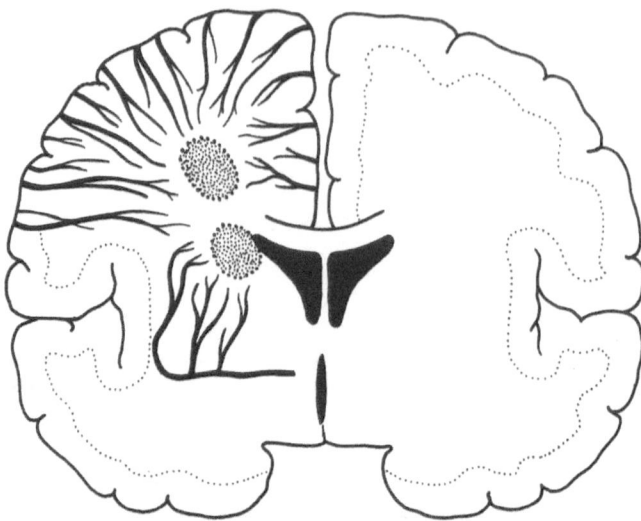

Fig. 8. Two typical lacunar cystic infarcts with presumed hemodynamic pathogenesis in the middle of the semioval center, where an area of vascular insufficiency exists in the terminal regions of the entire cortical supply of the anterior and upper middle cerebral arteries according to the theory of the most distant field, and a similar cystic lacunar (most distal field type) is seen in terminal areas of medial and lateral striate arteries

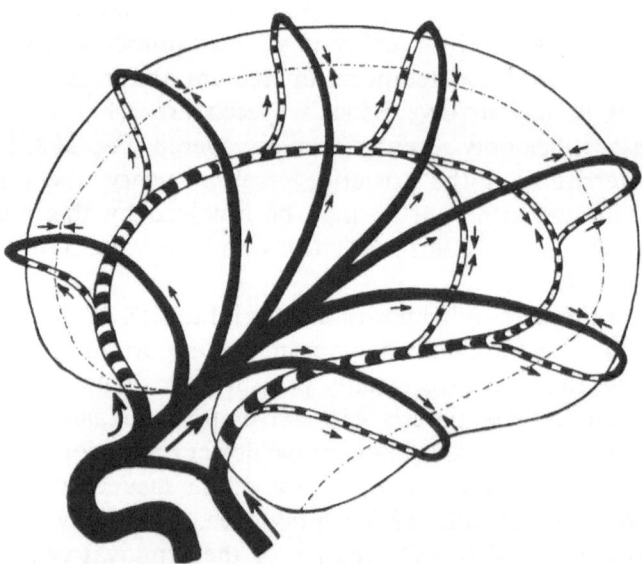

Fig. 9. The meningeal anastomoses (Heubner) form a reticulum on the upper surface of the brain between the three source arteries of each hemisphere

of pathogenesis contradicts somewhat the hypothesis of ZEUMER et al. (1981) that lacunar infarctions are usually the terminal defects of a branch going from the cortex down into the deep white matter (Fig. 37a).

The latter type of lacunar infarction, consistent with the most distant field concept, can be found in the territory of the anterior choroidal artery, located in the basal portion of the globus pallidus (Fig. 38a) or in the distal, terminal area of the lateral wall of the ventricular trigone (Fig. 39a). In this region infarctions apparently occur when the collateral flow from the medial posterior choroidal artery is insufficient (KLEIHUES 1966) and the anterior choroidal artery is occluded.

7. Differences in size and location of infarcts can be seen with occlusion of the same artery (Figs. 9, 10). This is most readily demonstrated with occlusion of the middle cerebral artery. Distal occlusion of the main trunk (Fig. 10) may produce one of the following:
a) A total infarct
b) A medium-sized infarct
c) A wedge-shaped infarct
d) A minimal infarct.

This is entirely dependent upon the amount of blood flow at the border zones of the middle cerebral artery territory, which may be sup-

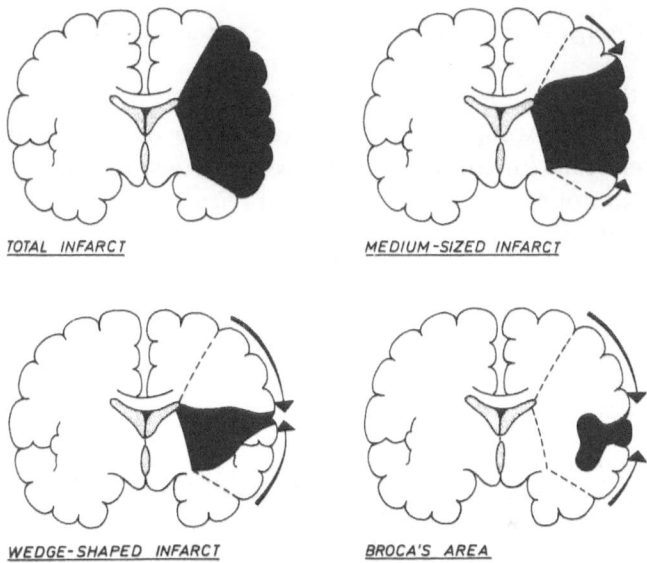

TOTAL INFARCT   MEDIUM-SIZED INFARCT

WEDGE-SHAPED INFARCT   BROCA'S AREA

Fig. 10. Various types and sizes of infarcts following specific hemodynamic patterns. Occlusion of the middle cerebral artery may be associated with either total infarct, medium-sized infarct, wedge-shaped infarct, or minimal infarct, depending upon the extent of collateral supply from the neighborhood

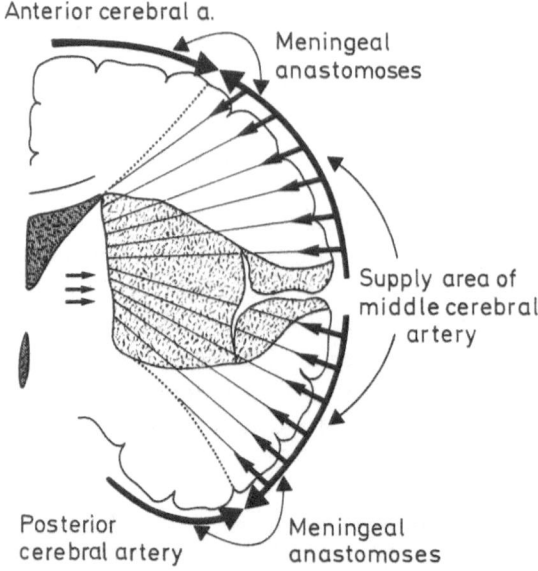

Fig. 11. A typical wedge-shaped infarct arising from hemodynamic insufficiency in the central part of the middle cerebral artery territory

plied by meningeal anastomoses from the anterior and posterior cerebral arteries.

Among the phenomena related to the hemodynamics of the collateral blood flow is the wedge-shaped infarct, which can easily be explained (Fig. 11) in occlusion of the middle cerebral artery since each branch of the anastomotic network probably supplies a segment of equal length in the territory of the middle cerebral artery. Of each segment one part can be superficial and the remainder deep after "perforating" the cortex. The longer the superficial segment of the particular artery and the more distant from the anastomotic supply, the shorter the perforating part will be.

3.2 The Hemorrhagic Type of Infarction
(Fig. 61 a, b)

We will discuss now why infarcts may become hemorrhagic. First, we note that pericapillary hemorrhages in the infarct present themselves mainly in the gray matter. This area has about five times more capillary volume and five times greater oxygen consumption than the white matter. Therefore, the cortex suffers first from cerebrovascular insufficiency, and the initial consequence may be greater permeability of the capillary walls.

In the following situations we can expect diapedetic hemorrhages in the gray matter:

1. If, for example, there is an intermittent medial temporal herniation producing a tentorial pressure cone. An intermittent hypoperfusion of the posterior cerebral artery may occur and cerebrovascular insufficiency in the medial part of the occipital lobe (Fig. 46a) will follow (ZÜLCH et al. 1974, Figs. 40 and 41)
2. If a vessel is occluded long enough to permit damage of the vascular endothelium and is then reopened (with a flow near the level of "survival grade" of brain tissue)
3. Probably – although this is not yet fully proven – in any case of cerebrovascular insufficiency near the threshold limit of 15% of normal circulation [OPITZ and SCHNEIDER (1950) rule of the degrees of cerebrovascular dysfunction and structural necrosis]
4. If an embolus disintegrates and blood flow is reestablished (hypothesis of the Boston school; C.M. FISHER 1951)
5. Following hypertensive crises where, statistically, infarcts are more frequently red (BOTTON 1955)
6. In the marginal zones of an anemic (white) infarct following establishment of collateral circulation (first described by VIRCHOW in the kidney).

Local hyperemia from "luxury perfusion" (CRONQVIST et al. 1975) can also appear similar to a hemorrhagic type of infarct in the CT scan. The aforementioned authors classified two-thirds of the infarcts in their series as ischemic and one-third as hemorrhagic.

The Patterns of Hemorrhagic Infarcts. The hemorrhagic infarct may:

1. Involve all of the infarcted cortex (Fig. 61a)
2. Be present only in the marginal zones, near collateral circulation
3. Be spotty, with preference for the base of the sulci.

Differential diagnosis between arterial hemorrhagic infarction and the venous type is possible on the basis of the location and the finer distribution of the hemorrhages. In arterial infarction, the hemorrhages are fine and thin and only faintly visible individually, and they occur exclusively in the cortex. Venous infarctions have single, slightly larger hemorrhages which are located mainly in the white matter, while the cortex is almost uninvolved.

The "hypertensive" hematomas occur predominantly in the putamen and may either remain localized (Fig. 62a) or extend into the neighboring white matter of the frontal, temporal, or parietal lobe (Fig. 62b). They may also rupture through the ventricular wall and introduce blood into the cerebro-spinal fluid (usually in the frontal horn).

Hypertensive hematomas may also occur in the thalamus and cerebellum (Fig. 62c). The latter are important because they (as well as some of those previously mentioned) are operable. Atypical hematomas (Fig. 62d) may occur elsewhere in younger persons and nonhypertensives.

The causes of decreased flow, the different types of acute and subacute vascular occlusions or stenoses, the disturbance of flow in the microcircula-tion, and other pertinent factors will not be discussed here (see ZÜLCH 1981, extensive description). However, as an introduction to the second chapter, which provides a systematic demonstration of individual CTs of infarcts, the data pertinent to the (technical) visualization of ischemic or edematous cerebral tissue in the CT scan need to be mentioned.

In summary, we want to emphasize that in spite of so many variables in the central and peripheral hemodynamics, differences in the vasculariza-tion of the cerebral tissue, complexity of the anastomoses and the resulting collateral circulations, and different rheological factors can often determine the location and extent of cerebrovascular insufficiency leading to an infarct. However, one must be well acquainted with the factors operative in the process of infarction.

Various types of "cardiovascular insufficiency" which may also pre-dispose to infarction will not be discussed in this work. However, the impor-tant work of REIN (1931, 1936), BÜCHNER (1939, 1964), and CORDAY and ROTHENBERG (1957), as well as the special contributions of OPITZ and SCHNEIDER (1950), must be mentioned.

4 Technical Aspects of Interpreting Computed Tomograms

A few of the more important principles are summarized here to facilitate interpretation in the following atlas of CTs. The topic, as we will see, is still surrounded by controversy. Due to the peculiarities of our series we were not able to test these differences, since serial tomograms or repetitive films could only rarely be taken in the course of the first six weeks. However, we mention the literature even when it does not correspond with our own experience.

4.1 Time Course of the Changes in Density of the Tissue

In focal cerebrovascular insufficiency the earliest change in some of the CT scans is seen after 3–8 h and is observed as a hypodense lesion (probably due to intracellular edema). In 50% of the cases changes are recognizable within the first 24 h, probably related to the additional formation of extracellular edema (ZÜLCH 1986). This percentage increases until the 3rd day. The longest time before any change is apparent has been said to be 10 days. However, as will be discussed later, this pattern can still change up to the 4th week (OSTERTAG and MUNDINGER 1978). In addition, the possibility of a change in tissue density produced by infusion of contrast medium (PULLICINO and KENDALL 1980) will be mentioned later.

In most cases the hypodense change due to edema is recognizable by the 2nd day (MASDEU et al. 1977; AULICH and FENSKE 1977; KOHLMEYER and GRASER 1978a, b; LEE et al. 1978; ALCALA et al. 1978; RADÜ and MOSELEY 1978; MÜLLER 1979).

4.2 Contrast Enhancement

Generally, an increase in density following infusion of contrast medium (enhancement) will be demonstrated beginning on the 5th day, with a further enhancement by the 2nd week which will peak by the 3rd week. By that time up to 95% of infarcts will be enhanced by contrast infusion.

WING et al. (1976) reported enhancement in 60% of infarcts in their series between the 2nd and 4th week, MASDEU et al. (1977) in 63%. These figures disagree with those of LEE et al. (1978), who found contrast enhancement in 88% of acute cases, and KAWASE et al. (1981), who observed contrast enhancement in more than 90% between the 10th day and the end of the 1st month. However, they did not continue their observations beyond the 2nd month. This is especially important because MASDEU et al. (1977) found contrast enhancement in 100% by the 3rd month. SKRIVER and OLSEN (1982) scanned 55 stroke patients at 3 days and after $2^1/_2$ weeks with and without contrast enhancement, and then again after 6 months without any contrast medium. They observed an absence of contrast enhancement during the first 3 days, and positive enhancement in 46% at $2^1/_2$ weeks. They concluded, therefore, that the most reproducible demonstration of infarction was a low CT scan density without enhancement, during the first 3 days after the stroke.

Sometimes extensive hyperemia of an infarcted area leads to a blush and intense contrast enhancement (in one-third of the cases between the 12th and 21st days; STEINHOFF et al. 1976). This is said to be caused by a breakdown of the blood-brain barrier.

HAYMAN et al. (1979) made the observation that contrast enhancement is more informative than a nonenhanced CT scan. HAMMER (1982) expressed great reluctance to infuse contrast medium into a patient with a suspected infarct for fear that an additional lesion might be produced.

The preceding data exemplify the differences of opinion encountered when one attempts critically to evaluate the available literature.

4.3 The Fogging Effect

A fogging effect in the CT has been described (BECKER et al. 1979) when an infarcted area is isodense (or nearly so) in the non enhanced scan, but is hyperdense after contrast enhancement [YOCK and MARSHALL 1975, between 10% and 20%; WING et al. 1976, 11%; NORTON et al. 1978, 13%; SKRIVER and OLSEN 1982, 54% (!)]. According to STEINHOFF and AMBROSE (1981), in some cases the initial lesions may be hypodense, changing to isodense and later becoming hypodense again.

AULICH et al. (1976) found a circumscribed hypodense lesion in only 6% during the first 2 days, but in 95% after the 1st week. ALCALÁ et al. (1978) observed that a primary hypodensity resulting from edema might change to isodensity after becoming hemorrhagic. It is evident that for exact diagnosis and verification of the ischemic damage serial studies are necessary, and that one must apply enhancement to the CT examination at each interval. This may not be possible and therefore for purposes of demonstrating an infarct one should adhere to the following rule: The first CT scan should be made on the 3rd day. If it is isodense, one should either apply contrast enhancement at that time or repeat the CT scan at a later date.

4.4 Increased Volume of the Tissue

When there is no change in the density of the compromised tissue, infarction may sometimes be recognized by the mass effect produced by edema. This is manifested by compression of the neighboring sulci and shift across the midline of parts of the ventricular system. These alterations may endure as long as 2–3 weeks. The edema formation may be very intense in some cases, e.g., in combined infarction in the territories of the anterior cerebral and the middle cerebral arteries (Fig. 27a), as seen in one of our cases (ZÜLCH 1968, Fig. 14a, b).

This increase in volume due to edema disappears after 8 weeks in 70%, according to MASDEU et al. (1977). Yet, as mentioned, a mass effect (Fig. 27a) from combined anterior cerebral and middle cerebral artery infarction can lead to a severe shift across the midline with herniation. This can be misleading, particularly when uncal herniation occurs contralateral to the infarcted area. Temporal lobe herniation due to tumor impinging on the posterior cerebral artery (ZÜLCH 1959; ZÜLCH et al. 1974, Figs. 40–42) can lead to medial occipital hemorrhagic infarction in the center of the supply area of the posterior cerebral artery (Fig. 46a) (ZÜLCH 1961, Figs. 41 and 42). However, there should not be any difficulty in the differential diagnosis of cerebrovascular and neoplastic processes (see HUBER et al. 1978).

More detailed information regarding differential diagnosis of infarcts by CT scan can be found in the monographs of VALK (1980) and KAZNER et al. (1981).

4.5 Protein-Rich Edema

Protein-rich edema may destroy myelin sheaths (ZÜLCH 1953, 1986). It has to be emphasized, however, that even massive edema may disappear without great damage to the myelin. This has been observed in one patient subsequent to hypertensive crisis (Fig. 63a, b). Prognosis will vary depending on whether or not there is destruction of myelin (see also RAIL and PERKIN 1980).

4.6 Improper Prognosis

The problem of improper prognosis based on CT scan is illustrated by one of my cases of middle cerebral artery territory infarctions with contralateral palsy which was more marked in the upper extremity. Because of the extensive middle cerebral cortical infarction as seen on CT (Fig. 64a), the prognosis was said to be poor. However, after 3 months, the patient had only a slight residual hemiparesis with movements preserved at all joints. Even the fingers were able to make independent movements. On the other hand, after 3 months the CT scan was still suggestive of cortical necrosis predominantly in the medial and basal parts of the territory of the middle cerebral artery. The neurological examination after 6 months showed almost no motor signs, although marked abnormalities such as visual amnesia and focal epileptic seizures were present. To our surprise the CT scan (Fig. 64b) was still basically identical to the first picture, which was suggestive of gross necrosis.

4.7 Relating a Focal Lesion to a Transient Ischemic Attack

The problem of relating a focal lesion to a transient ischemic attack (TIA) is not resolved. On at least two occasions we have observed a slightly hypodense zone 1–2 days after such an event. According to the literature this may be seen in 25% of cases within that time period. On the other hand, TIA caused by small lacunar lesions may be accompanied by complete clinical recovery.

4.8 Flow Measurements

One final point that needs to be discussed is the question of whether flow measurements after enhancement can be evaluated in order to show the site of cerebrovascular insufficiency. It seemed to us from our initial experience that "dynamic computed tomography" permitted comparison and measurement of identical fields of interest on both sides in order to establish a relationship between the serial CT pattern and prognosis (TRAUPE et al. 1979). This idea, however, must be reexamined.

II Correlations of CT Scan Patterns with Pathoanatomical Specimens

The present chapter aims to compare the infarct as observed in the CT scan with the pathoanatomical appearance at autopsy, in an attempt to obtain more information regarding pathogenesis. Our interpretation of the pathogenesis of infarcts is based on almost 25 years of experience with cerebral angiography and clinical morphological observation in such cases (described in detail in the textbooks by KAUTZKY et al. 1982 and by ZÜLCH 1981).

The second part of this correlated study has one drawback. It is based on a series of approximately 800 anatomical specimens of infarcts, the majority of which were collected before the establishment of the intensive care unit within our neurological department and in the pre-CT-scan era. Therefore, it has been impossible to correlate the less common pictures with individual clinical observations. Furthermore, most of the anatomical specimens had been sliced by coronal section, making it necessary to "reconstruct" the CT scans mentally into coronal slices.

It should be emphasized, however, that:
1. Most of the published work concerned with the pathology and pathogenesis of infarction has been based on coronal slices.
2. In fact, coronal slicing has facilitated the understanding of the hemodynamics of infarction. This can clearly be seen in publications over the past 50 years.
3. Correlation is feasible between an anteroposterior angiogram and the coronal slice of the specimen but not so readily with a horizontal slice.
4. NMR is usually also showing coronal slices and angiograms by DSA will be frequent in the future.

We have classified approximately 1000 CTs with infarcts, of which 56% were in the left hemisphere. The following gross localization (for a topographical sketch of the most important regions mentioned in the text, see Fig. 66) was noted (Figs. 12 and 13):

Middle cerebral artery	27%	Opercular	3%
Posterior cerebral artery	12%	Wedge-shaped	3%
Lacunar	12%	Pons	3%
Caudate	10%	Cerebellar (dorsal and ventral)	3%
Internal capsule	5%	Anterior cerebral artery	2%
Three-territory border	5%	Peduncular	2%
Multiple	4%	Long central artery	1%
Thalamus	4%	(recurrent artery of Heubner)	
Bilateral	3%	Pure watershed circular infarcts	1%

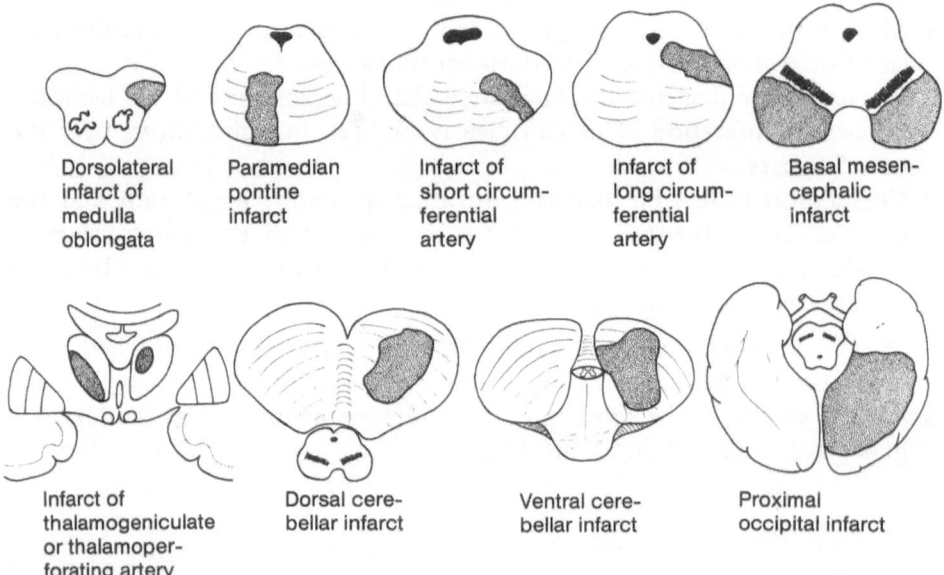

Fig. 12. Schematic view of the principal types of infarcts within the territory of the internal carotid artery (see Chap. III)

Dorsolateral infarct of medulla oblongata	Paramedian pontine infarct	Infarct of short circumferential artery	Infarct of long circumferential artery	Basal mesencephalic infarct

Infarct of thalamogeniculate or thalamoperforating artery	Dorsal cerebellar infarct	Ventral cerebellar infarct	Proximal occipital infarct

Fig. 13. Schematic view of the principal types of infarcts within the territory of the vertebrobasilar system

III The Systematic Classification of Brain Infarcts

1 Carotid Territory

1.1 Superficial Infarcts in the Territory of the Middle Cerebral Artery

1.1.1 Infarcts of the Middle Cerebral Artery

1.1.1.1 Complete Infarct of the Middle Cerebral Artery Including the Striate and Anterior Choroidal Arteries (Fig. 14a, b)

Total infarction of the supply area of the middle cerebral artery, including the anterior choroidal artery, does not always occur following occlusion of the middle cerebral artery. We know from our early experience (ZÜLCH and HERBERG 1949) that following acute occlusion of the internal carotid artery in the neck, infarction occurred in two-thirds of the cases, corresponding to the complete, or at least the central, territory of the middle cerebral artery. This has been confirmed by RADÜ and MOSELEY (1978), who found infarcts following occlusion of the carotid artery in 21 out of 35 cases.

Complete infarction of the territory of the middle cerebral artery is relatively rare compared to other types of infarction. The four predilection sites of occlusion of the middle cerebral arteries are depicted in Fig. 65 as derived from our own angiographic experience (KAUTZKY et al. 1976, 1982). Occlusions in location III lead most often to complete infarction of the supply area; those in location I cause infarction near the "stump," while those in location IV often produce a striatal, opercular, or insular infarct.

Cortical lesions observed in the CT scan can be divided into three groups, namely the anterior, the middle, and the posterior infarcts of the middle cerebral artery. These types of infarction are explained by occlusion of either the anterior, the middle, or the posterior group of sylvian arteries (according to the pattern of the "candelabra"; see SALAMON and HUANG 1976, Fig. 70b, d) or as a consequence of insufficient collateral circulation either anteriorly or posteriorly through leptomeningeal anastomoses (Fig. 9) when the middle cerebral artery is totally occluded (this has been discussed above, see p. 8 ff.).

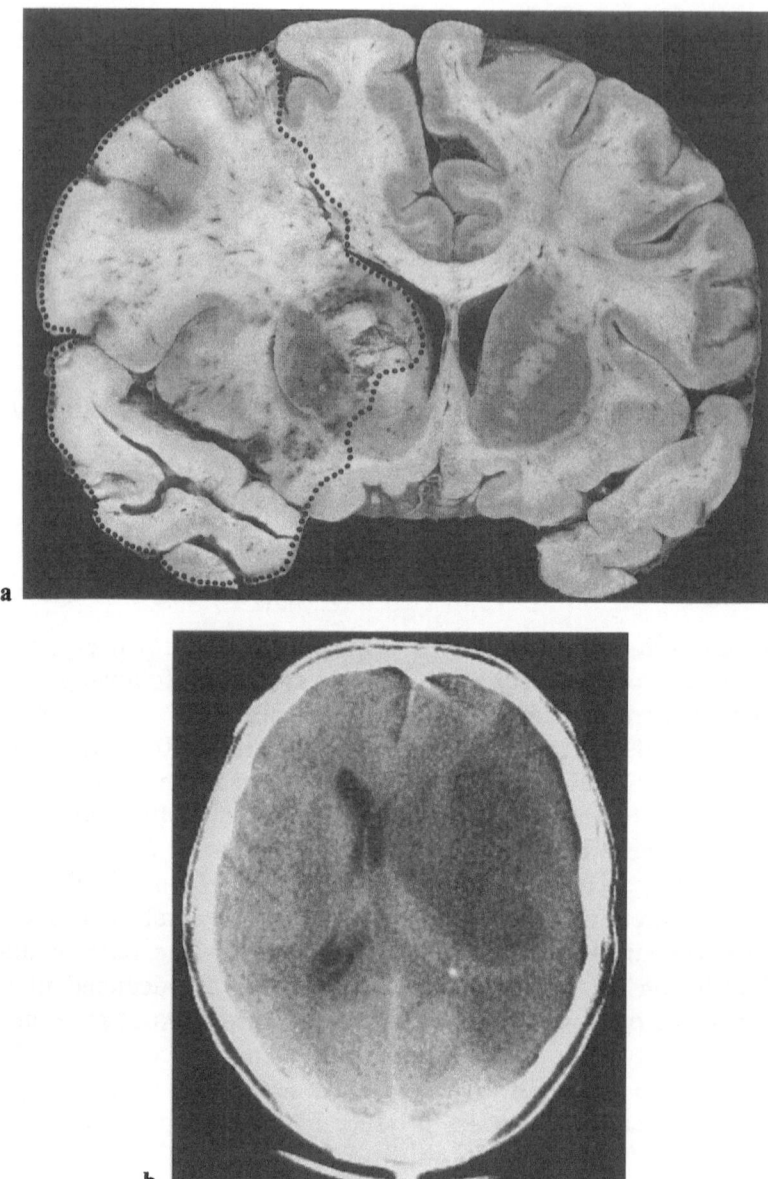

Fig. 14. a Complete infarct of middle cerebral artery including the striate arteries. The infarct is near the border of the anterior cerebral artery territory and is partly hemorrhagic. **b** Complete infarct of middle cerebral artery, including branches to basal ganglia. Due to considerable edema formation, there is a shift toward the contralateral side with compression of the lateral ventricle

Just as one can find a subdivision of the infarct types in a rostral/caudal direction, a subdivision in the lateral projection also exists. In these cases one finds either a merely cortical lesion, since the basal ganglia are supplied by the striate and choroidal arteries, or a deep infarct (see p. 22, Fig. 12).

1.1.1.2 Infarct of the Middle Cerebral Artery Excluding the Striate Arteries (Fig. 15a, b)

If the lesion in the middle cerebral artery is located beyond the origin of the striate arteries (Fig. 65 IV), a purely cortical infarct with sparing of the striatum and pallidum will ensue when the distal branches of the candelabra are not sufficiently supplied by the meningeal anastomoses with the neighboring arteries.

1.1.1.3 Infarct of the Middle Cerebral Artery, Anterior Third (Fig. 16a, b)

This type of infarct in the territory of the middle cerebral artery is one of the most common. Its frequency can possibly be explained by the different subdivision patterns of the candelabra stem (see SALAMON and HUANG 1976, pp. 84–85, Fig. 70b, d) proximal to the takeoff of the precentral artery. The infarcted territory corresponds approximately to that of the prefrontal and the central arteries of the candelabra system (Fig. 67). A hemodynamic explanation might also be possible by virtue of different actions of the meningeal anastomoses.

An investigation by WODARZ (1975) related to our series of cases of middle cerebral artery branch occlusions has not provided any information about the above-mentioned types of pathogenesis. He found a higher frequency of branch occlusions only in the parietotemporal area as well as with associated occlusions of the anterior and posterior parietal and the posterior temporal arteries.

1.1.1.4 Infarct of the Middle Cerebral Artery, Middle Third (Fig. 17a, b)

Infarction of the middle third of the middle cerebral artery territory is also relatively frequent. It encompasses the territory of the anterior precentral and anterior central arteries, sometimes including the anterior branches of the anterior parietal artery. It seems possible that the pathogenesis of this type of infarct may be a combined occlusion of the above-mentioned arteries – similar to that observed with infarction in the anterior third. If this is so, then the location of the infarct could be explained by the subdivisions of the candelabra (see SALAMON and HUANG 1976, Fig. 70b, d). Yet it appears more likely that it adheres to a hemodynamic pattern related to flow from meningeal anastomoses operating anteriorly and posteriorly. The size and location of these infarcts is variable, with the borders

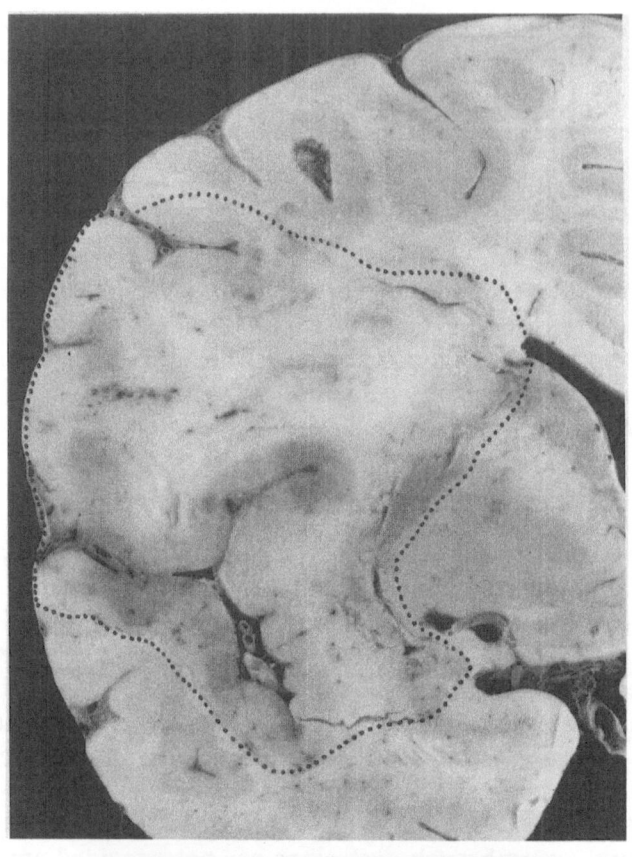

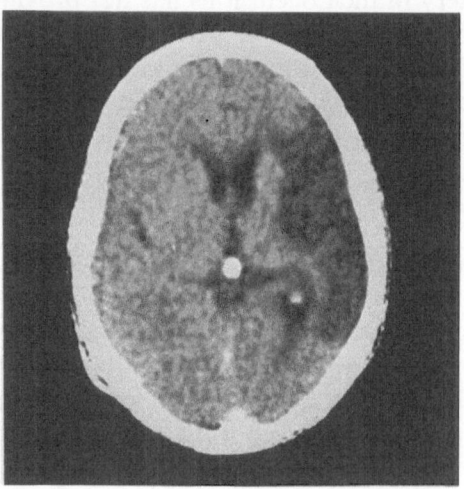

Fig. 15. a Near complete infarct of middle cerebral artery excluding striate arteries.
b Near complete infarct of middle cerebral artery, sparing arteries to basal ganglia.
Since infarct is old, frontal horn is dilated

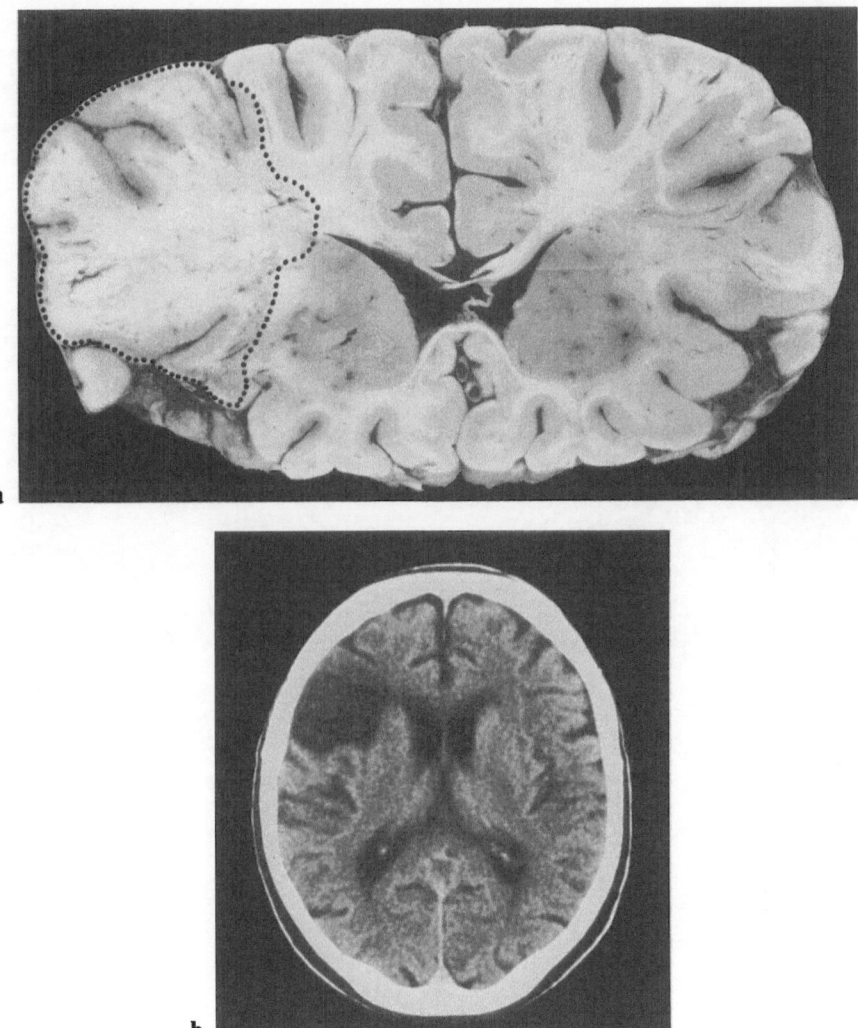

Fig. 16. a Complete infarct of anterior third of the middle cerebral artery territory.
b Infarct of anterior third of middle cerebral artery territory

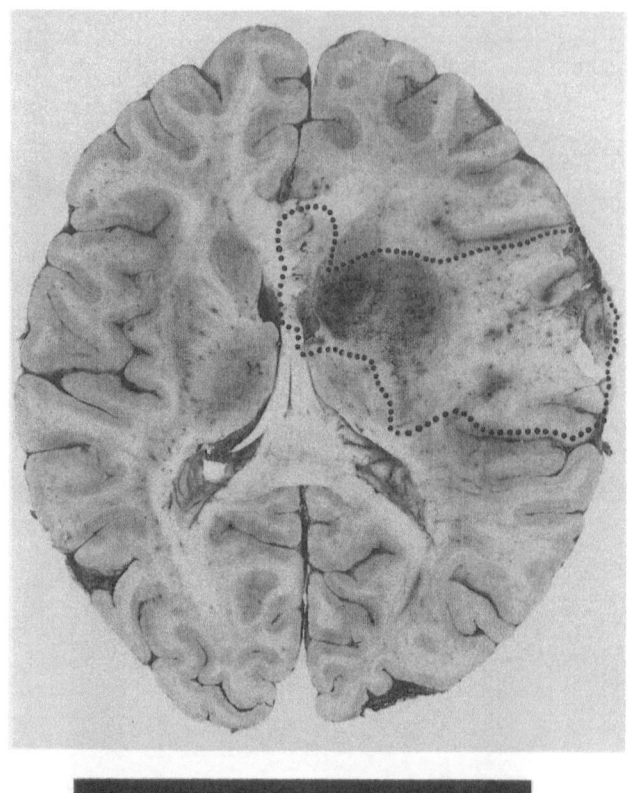

a

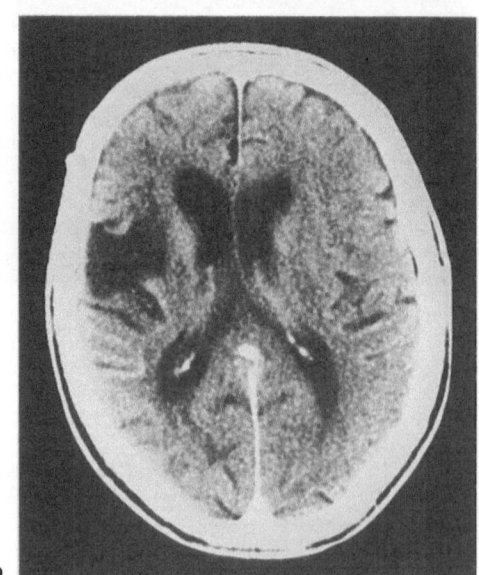

b

Fig. 17a, b. Infarct in middle third of middle cerebral artery, including striate arteries

extending either rostrally, caudally, dorsally, or ventrally. We have seen examples of all of these locations without any direct relation to specific branches of the sylvian group (Fig. 67). This fact would add more support for hemodynamic variability, as does the fact that we have seen infarcts of the middle third with total infarction of the basal ganglia below and other infarcts of the same arterial area without involvement of the striate arteries.

1.1.1.5 Infarct of the Middle Cerebral Artery, Posterior Third (Fig. 18a, b)

As with the first two groups of middle cerebral artery infarcts, one can attempt to explain this type not only from the subdivision of the candelabra, but also from hemodynamic patterns. In these cases the supply areas of the anterior and posterior parietal arteries and the artery of the angular gyrus are compromised and, eventually, parts of the territory of the occipito-temporal artery as well. The supply area of the latter artery is depicted by SALAMON and HUANG (1976, p. 86) as covering the entire convex surface of the occipital lobe, but this location contradicts the experience of most observers.

1.1.1.6 Four Special Types of Infarct Within the Territory of the Middle Cerebral Artery

Wedge-Shaped Infarct (Fig. 19a, b). This triangular infarct deep within the hemisphere, the apex of which points to the cortex, cannot be explained by the Cohnheim principle. This type is common and we have observed a large number of such infarcts both as anatomic specimens and in CT scans.

The wedge-shaped infarct is recognizable grossly on the surface only by a deep groove within the cortex. It comprises predominantly the deep inner territories of the middle cerebral artery and the inner parts of the opercula, and leaves the striatum uninvolved. We have attempted to explain this curious pattern by a schematic drawing (ZÜLCH 1981, Fig. 134, p. 137). Validation of this explanation has been presented already on p. 14, Fig. 11.

Opercular Infarct (Fig. 20a, b). This type of infarct is situated predominantly in the frontal operculum and usually touches the upper edge of the insula. It is very common and stereotyped. We have observed it just as frequently in CT scans as in anatomical specimens. It corresponds both in its pathogenesis and its limited extent to a "minimal" infarction of the supply area of the middle cerebral artery (see p. 13, Fig. 10), or to the anterior half of the "center" of the territory.

It should be noted that it is very often hemorrhagic, which would indicate that it is caused by cerebrovascular insufficiency near the "critical border"

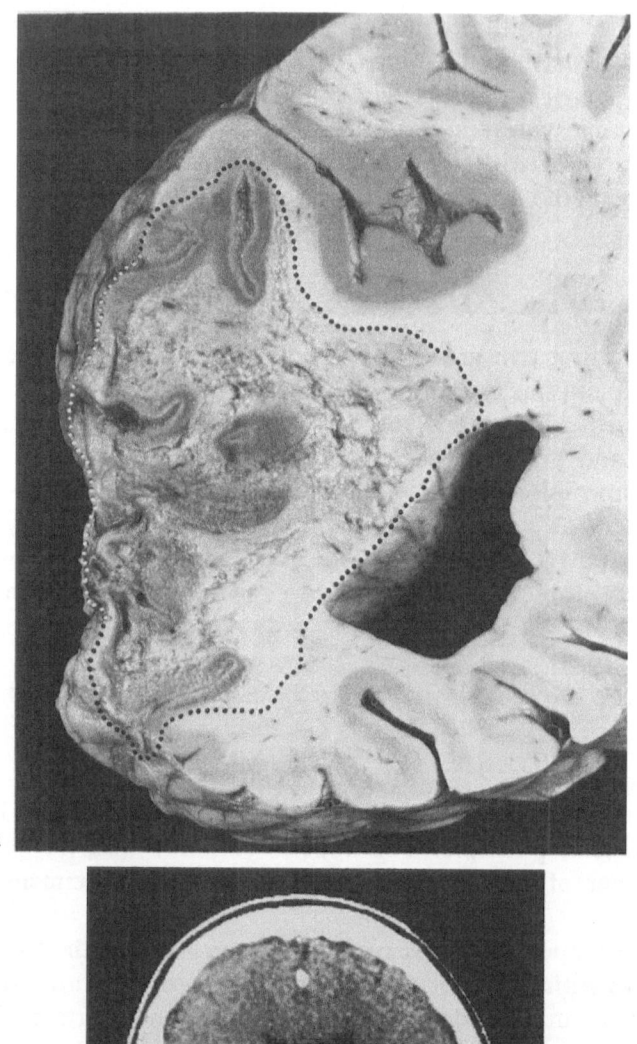

a

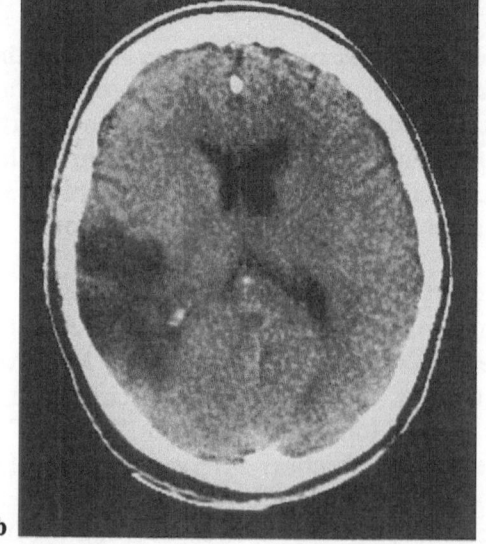

b

Fig. 18. a Partly cystic infarct in posterior third of middle cerebral artery territory.
b Infarct in posterior third of middle cerebral artery territory

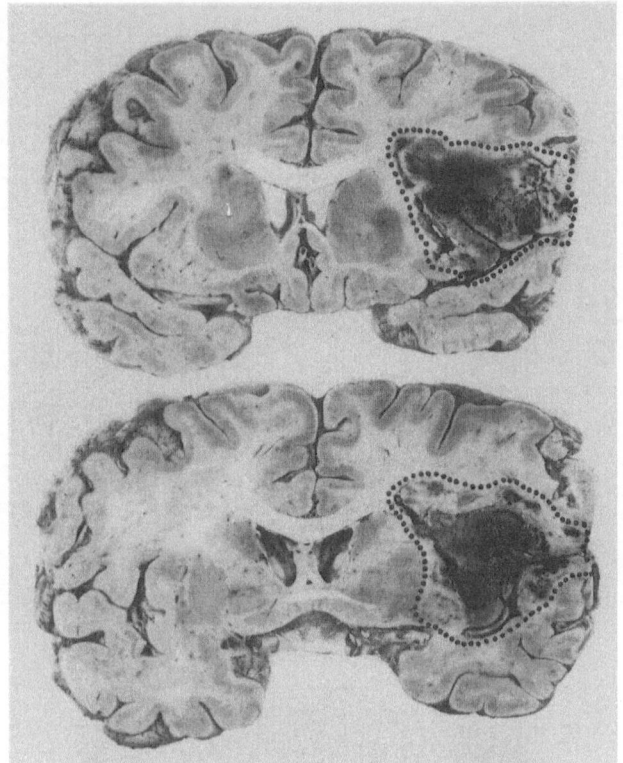

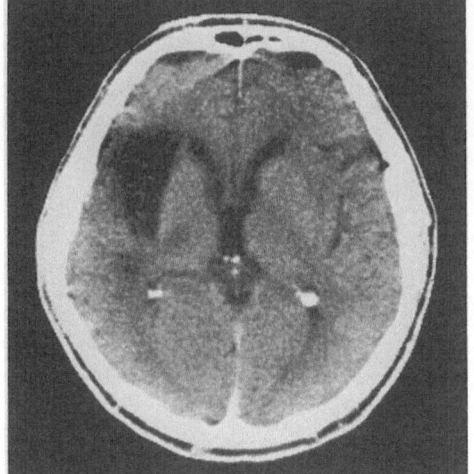

Fig. 19. a Typical fresh hemorrhagic wedge-shaped infarct. **b** Wedge-shaped infarct in supply area of middle cerebral artery

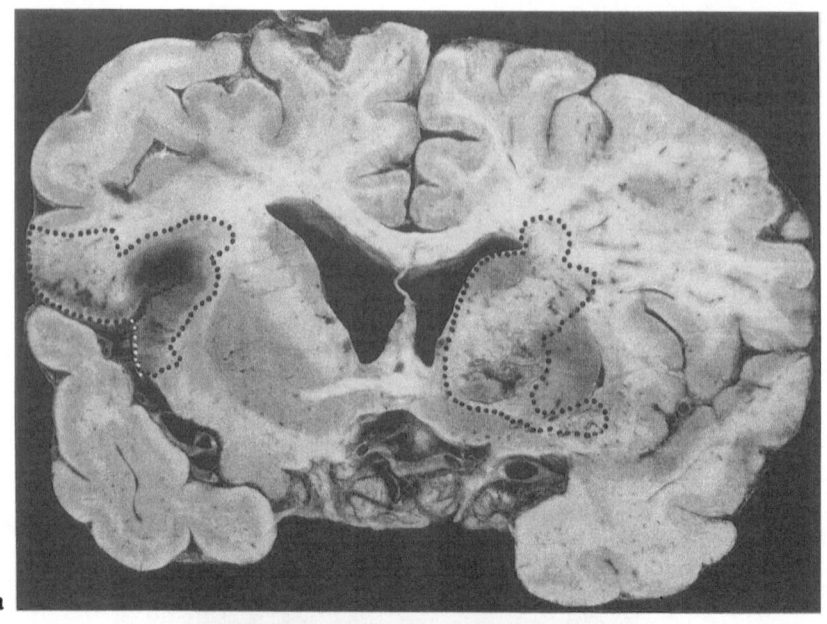

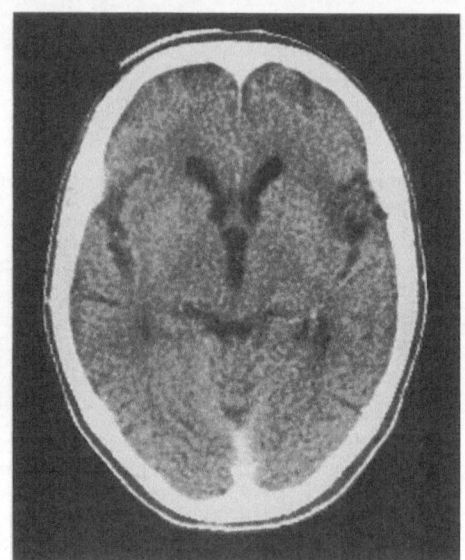

Fig. 20. a *Left*, typical infarct in frontal operculum, extending to insula. *Right*, infarct in caudatum medial peak of pallidum and neighboring internal capsule. **b** Infarct in frontal operculum extending into cortex and subcortex of insula

(see hemorrhagic infarct, p. 14). If situated on the left side, it may explain many transient ischemic attacks occurring as expressive aphasia, a clinical presentation which is so common in the elderly. It may also produce a facial droop (see also p. 11, Figs. 7, 20).

Insular Infarcts. Insular infarcts must be partial infarcts of the deep supply area of the middle cerebral artery. The cortex and the subcortex are not infrequently involved along with the frontal operculum, so that both regions may be compromised.

Infarct in the Center of the Territory of the Middle Cerebral Artery (Fig. 21a, b). This type of infarct was described as a concept during our early attempts (Fig. 5c) to understand the hemodynamics of infarction (ZÜLCH 1961, Fig. 41). The anterior part of this central area of cerebrovascular insufficiency was recognized at that time in pathological specimens as it is now in CT scans (see p. 25). However, the surprisingly frequent occurrence of similar processes in the elderly (as observed in the CT scan) in the posterior part of the insula (hypodensity, enlargement of sulci) could only be explained by a more posteriorly located hemodynamic insufficiency. The latter compromised the temporal and parietal operculum and the underlying insular convolutions. It often presented itself bilaterally and with changes of different severity.

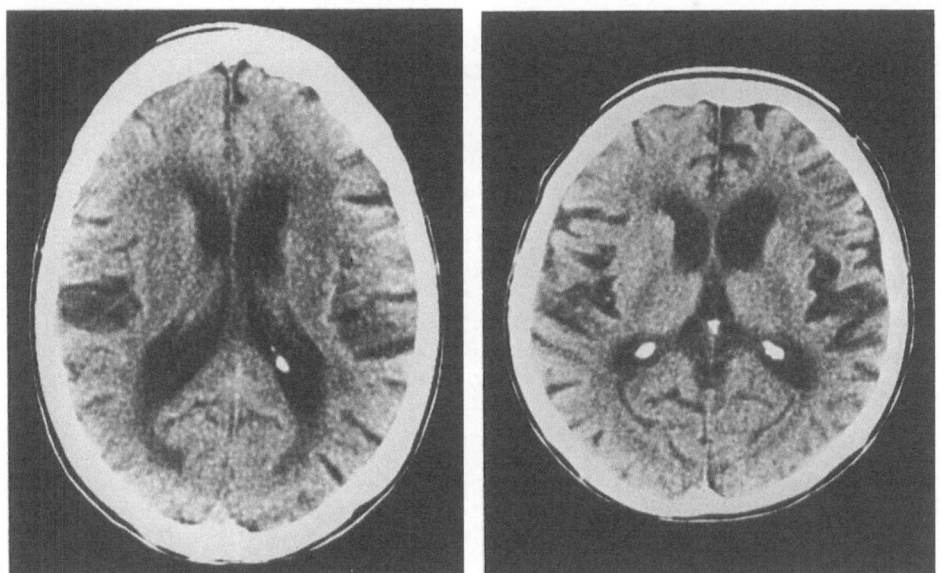

a   b

Fig. 21a, b. Infarct in the center of the supply area of the middle cerebral artery

1.1.1.7 Spotty Infarcts of the Territory of the Middle Cerebral Artery

Frequently, spotty infarcts appear in the depths of the area of supply of the middle cerebral artery. They probably originate as a result of a hemodynamic principle similar to that of some of the infarcts described above, where the collateral flow is variable. Depending upon the nature of the defect in central hemodynamics and the size of the meningeal anastomoses, a critical area of ischemia can occur in different locations such as in the inner part of the temporal operculum, in the insular region, or elsewhere in the supply area of the middle cerebral artery.

1.1.1.8 Bilateral Infarcts of the Middle Cerebral Artery

Bilateral infarction in the supply area of the middle cerebral artery is not so rare, although the two infarcts usually have a different time of origin (Fig. 22). One can find, for instance, on one side an infarct-cyst and on the other side a hemorrhagic infarct of more recent origin. The type of infarct follows one of the already described patterns.

It is important clinically that in this type of bilateral infarction cortical deafness may arise, as was observed in one of our cases (see also ADAMS et al. 1977; EARNEST et al. 1977). If the frontal operculum or the F-3 convolution on both sides is compromised, a total loss of speech may ensue (LEVINE and MOHR 1979).

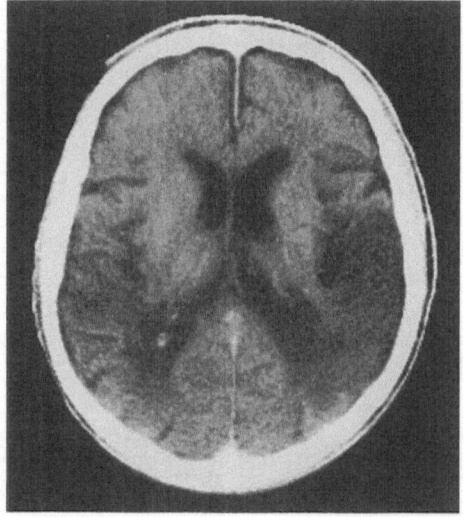

Fig. 22. Bilateral infarction of the middle cerebral artery

1.1.1.9 Subcortical Infarct in the Territory of the Middle Cerebral Artery
(Fig. 23 a, b)

We have not been able to clarify the pathogenesis of gross subcortical ischemic lesions observed in the depth of the supply area of this artery, as shown in the pictures. Neither have we been able to establish the pathogenesis from the clinical data, although this type of infarct is not uncommon in our CT series.

It is possible that subsequent severe edema in the white matter of the hemisphere (see Fig. 63 a, b with edema following a hypertensive crisis) could cause such an anatomical lesion.

In our observations the area of infarction could reach the ventricular wall, but it never involved the cortex. A pathogenetic pattern similar to that of the wedge-shaped infarcts (see Fig. 11), yet involving only the deeper parts of the white matter, would be feasible (see p. 14).

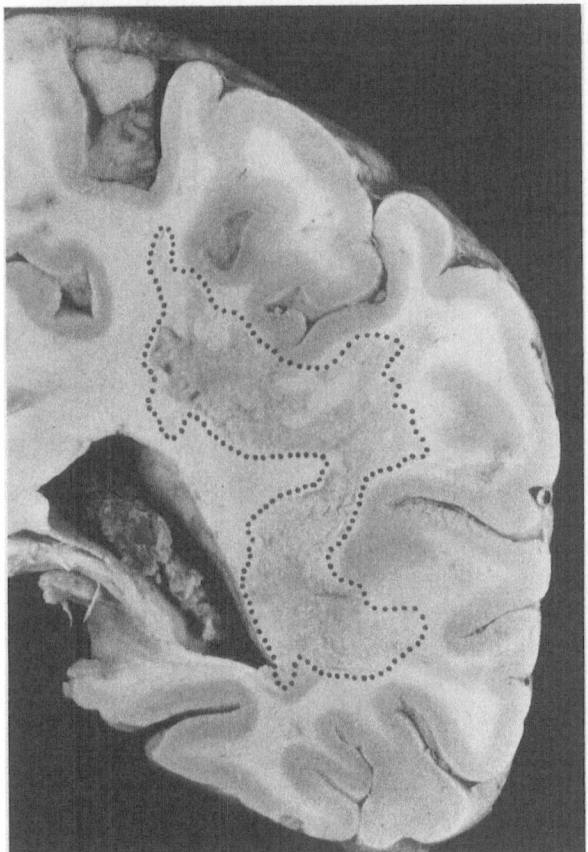
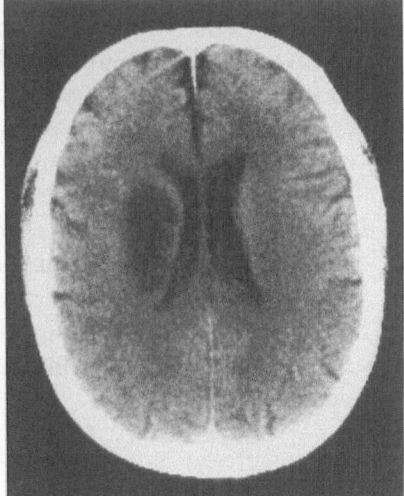

a b

Fig. 23. a Large infarct in subcortex extending to wall of trigone. **b** Large infarct in subcortex of middle third of middle cerebral artery territory

1.1.2 Infarcts in the Anterior Cerebral Artery Territory
(Figs. 24a, b, and 25a, b)

Infarcts of the anterior cerebral artery are more often irregularly extended and more often difficult to explain pathogenetically than those of the middle cerebral artery because of the unreliable collateral supply through meningeal anastomoses. Not only are the meningeal anastomoses less clearly defined, but they are less regularly formed, as we have noted in the middle cerebral artery territory. For instance, the interhemispheric communication of the two anterior cerebral arteries above the corpus callosum (ZÜLCH 1981, Fig. 14) is by no means a regularly occurring communication, and this is also true for the anastomoses along the corpus callosum (FISCHER-BRÜGGE 1949; see also KAUTZKY et al. 1976, 1982, Fig. 134), which are unreliable in their function, as is well known by most authors working in the field of angiography. The collateral blood supply comes from the posterior cerebral artery and runs anteriorly above the corpus callosum into the supply area of the anterior cerebral artery. This anastomosis is frequently visible in angiograms of the vertebrobasilar circulation when there is insufficiency in the anterior cerebral artery system. The gyrus cinguli, in particular, and some more anteriorly situated parts of the territory of the anterior cerebral artery are irrigated through this anastomosis. The spotty appearance of the infarct may be the consequence of these variable anastomotic patterns.

1.1.2.1 Infarcts of the Anterior Cerebral Artery, Anterior Division
(Fig. 24a, b)

Infarcts in the anterior division of the anterior cerebral artery will commonly involve the frontal pole with a predilection for the medial parts supplied by the orbitofrontal and frontopolar arteries and possibly also the internal anterior frontal artery. It must be emphasized, however, that these massive, readily recognized infarcts in the territory of the anterior cerebral artery are uncommon, because of an adequate collateral supply. This is due to the presence of numerous interconnections between the meningeal anastomoses of the anterior and middle cerebral arteries, as well as between the two anterior cerebral arteries themselves through the anterior communicating artery and the previously described transverse anastomoses above the corpus callosum. The gyrus cinguli and the half of the corpus callosum of the corresponding hemisphere may be spared because of these anastomoses.

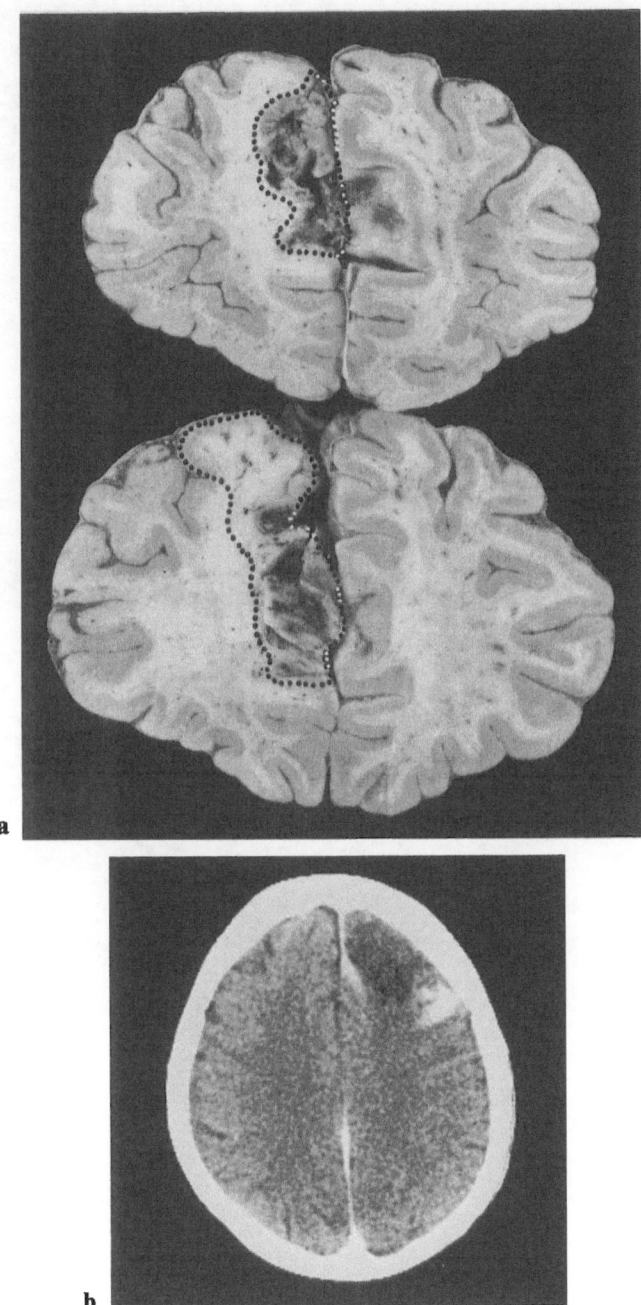

Fig. 24. a Partial infarct of anterior third of anterior cerebral artery area, partly extending to opposite side. **b** Infarct in anterior third of middle cerebral artery territory with hemorrhagic margins

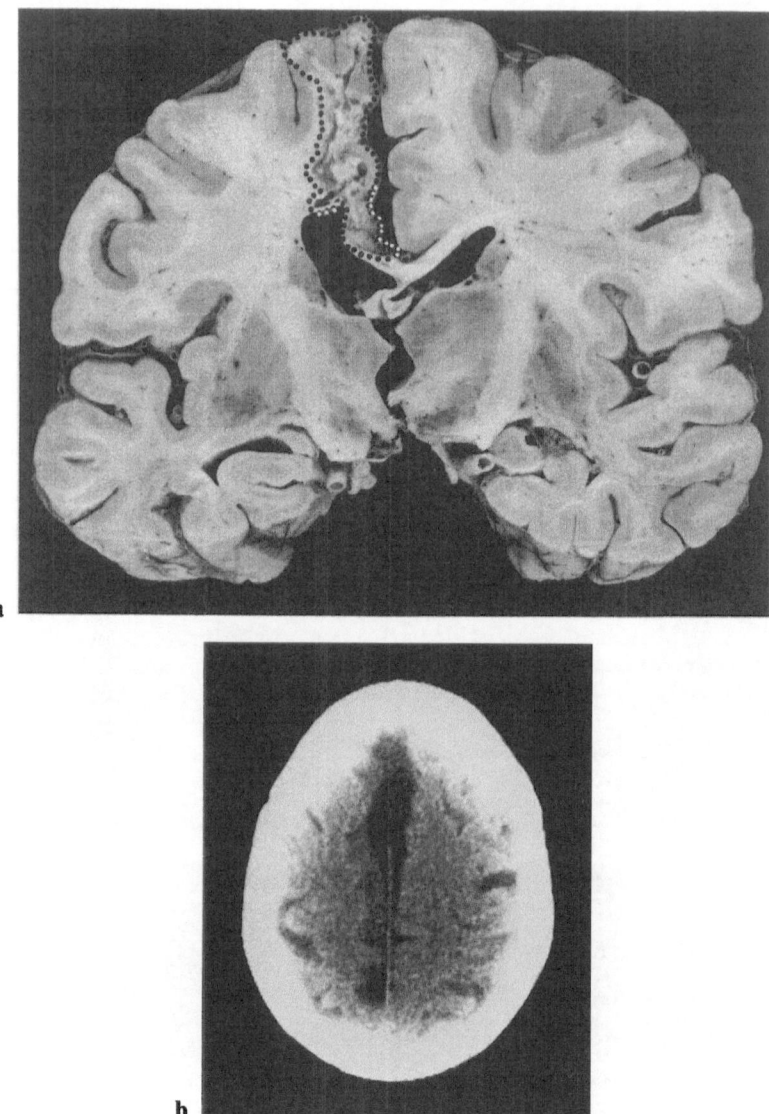

Fig. 25. a Old cystic, formerly ischemic, total infarct in anterior division of anterior cerebral artery. Enlargement of cella media. **b** Right-sided infarct in medial division of anterior cerebral artery

1.1.2.2 Infarcts of the Anterior Cerebral Artery, Posterior Division
(Fig. 25 a, b)

The territory of the posterior division of the anterior cerebral artery is rarely involved by infarction, since with involvement of the anterior division the anastomoses above the corpus callosum (FISCHER-BRÜGGE 1949) will supply the territory of the posterior division. Infarction occurs only when this meningeal anastomosis is less well formed or is not present at all, or if the vertebrobasilar system itself is not able to contribute to the circulation. When these infarcts occur, they have a partly spotty arrangement. The gyrus cinguli may be the first to be spared because of its direct blood supply through the corpus callosum anastomosis.

1.1.2.3 Total Infarction of the Anterior Cerebral Artery Territory

Since, as already described, the anterior division of the anterior cerebral artery is well supplied by anastomoses, total infarction of the supply area of the anterior cerebral artery is a rarity. It usually occurs if, in addition to the local lesion, there is a combined central hemodynamic disturbance, and then it may be combined with total infarction of the middle cerebral artery (Fig. 27 a, b) (see p. 41).

1.1.2.4 Spotty Infarcts in the Anterior Cerebral Artery Territory

We have emphasized above how variable the collateral blood supply is through the anterior communicating artery, which serves as a transverse anastomosis between the two anterior cerebral arteries; moreover, the anastomosis across the corpus callosum is also variable. Yet, additional circulation through meningeal anastomoses from the middle cerebral artery and posterior cerebral artery is relatively constant. As a result of these multiple possibilities for collateral circulation with their different degrees of function, spotty infarcts are not uncommon.

1.1.2.5 Infarcts in the Territory of the Long Central Artery
(Recurrent Artery of Heubner)
(Fig. 26 a, b)

When frontally situated infarcts in anterior cerebral artery territory are classified, one will observe peculiar, usually cystic infarcts, in the medial supraorbital convolutions and the neighboring parts of the corresponding striatum. These are caused by occlusion of the long central artery (recurrent artery of Heubner) (ZÜLCH 1981, Fig. 153). This artery originates, with only a few exceptions (1%), from the anterior cerebral artery. As a rule, this rare infarct is smaller than the actual supply area of the artery (KRIBS and KLEIHUES 1971; EINSIEDEL-LECHTAPE and KLEIHUES 1977).

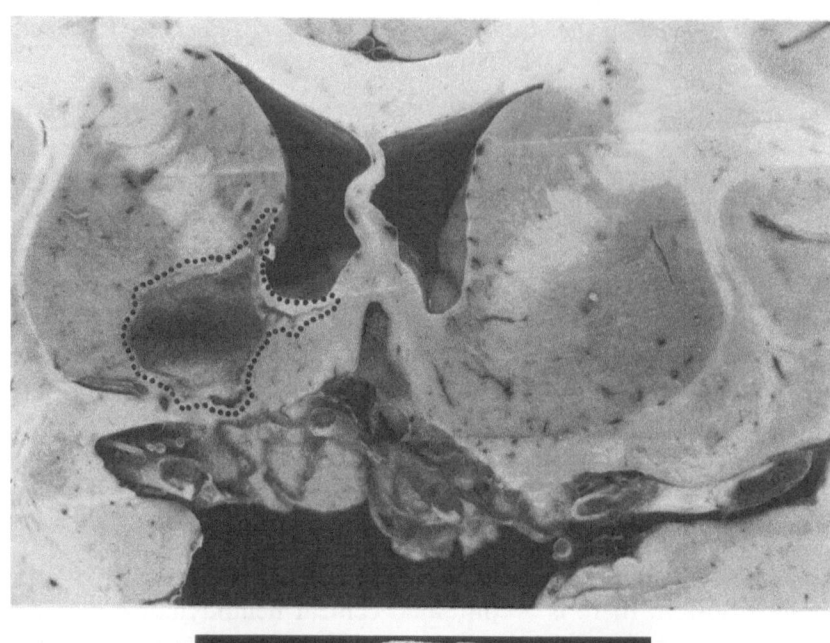

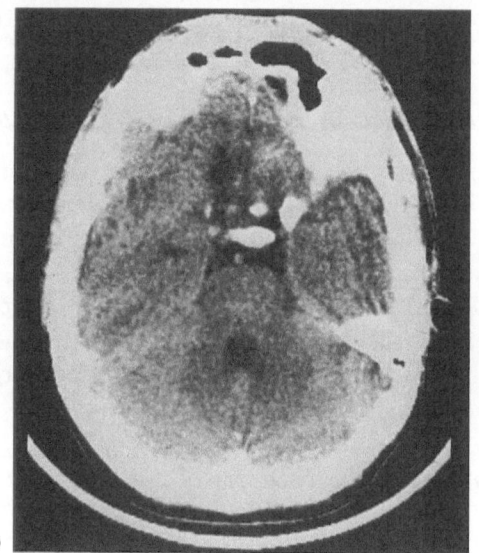

Fig. 26. a Old cystic infarct in irrigation area of right long central artery (recurrent artery of Heubner). **b** Infarct in basal supply area of long central artery (recurrent artery of Heubner)

1.1.3 Combined Infarcts

Infarcts occurring at the same time or alternately in the territories of several large arteries are not unusual. We know all about theoretically possible combinations of occlusions which produce infarcts in the supply territory of the internal carotid artery and that of the vertebrobasilar system. However, there are some combinations which occur more frequently than others.

1.1.3.1 Combined Infarcts of the Anterior and Middle Cerebral Artery Territories (Fig. 27a, b)

This combined infarct involves the major parts of one hemisphere. When both occur simultaneously (Fig. 27a, b), life may be endangered because of severe edema which may ensue, especially if both infarcts are hemorrhagic (ZÜLCH 1981, Fig. 154a, b). When this occurs, the increase in cerebral volume due to edema is so great that a shift in the medial portion of the temporal lobe toward the contralateral side produces pressure on the cerebral peduncle at the sharp margin of the tentorium. This causes entrapment of the peduncle with contralateral symptomatology often leading to an angiographic study of the "wrong side" (KAUTZKY et al. 1976, 1982).

1.1.3.2 Combined Infarcts of the Middle and Posterior Cerebral Arteries (Fig. 28a, b)

These combined infarcts can occur simultaneously or at different times, involving either one hemisphere (Fig. 29a) or both hemispheres.

1.1.4 Total Infarcts of the Internal Carotid Artery Territory (Fig. 29b)

When the internal carotid artery is occluded and the collateral supply by the many potential anastomoses fails to operate, a general hemodynamic insufficiency is created. When this occurs, the "total" supply area may be infarcted, as described above. Since in 20% of the general population the posterior cerebral artery has its origin from the carotid artery, its territory may also be included and thereby produce infarction of the entire hemisphere (Fig. 29b).

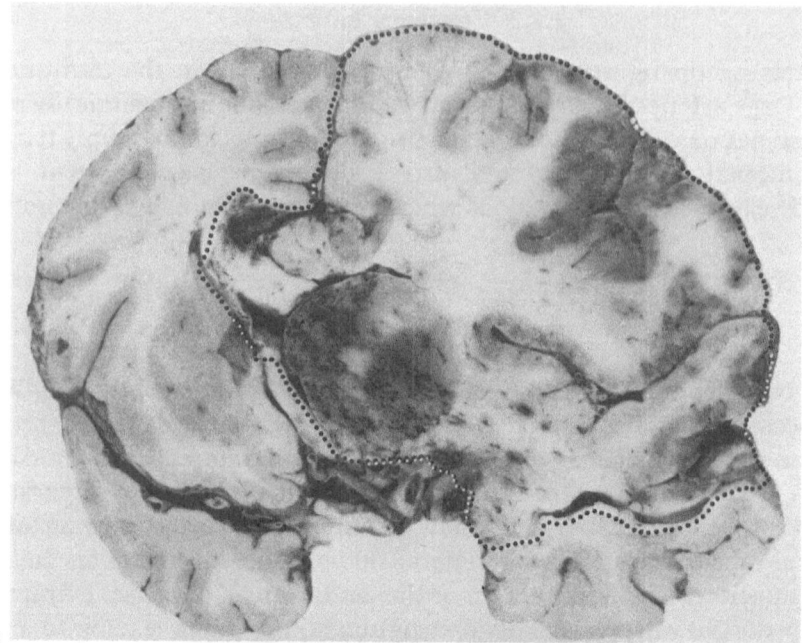

a

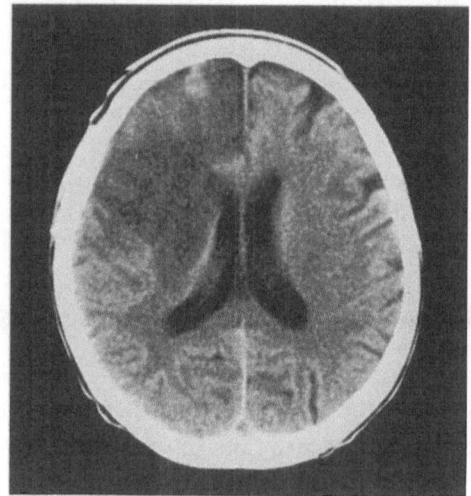

b

Fig. 27. a Massive fresh hemorrhagic infarction of the middle cerebral artery in combination with infarct of the anterior cerebral artery, which is grossly filled with edema and shows considerable shift to opposite side. **b** Combined total infarct of the anterior and semitotal of middle cerebral arteries

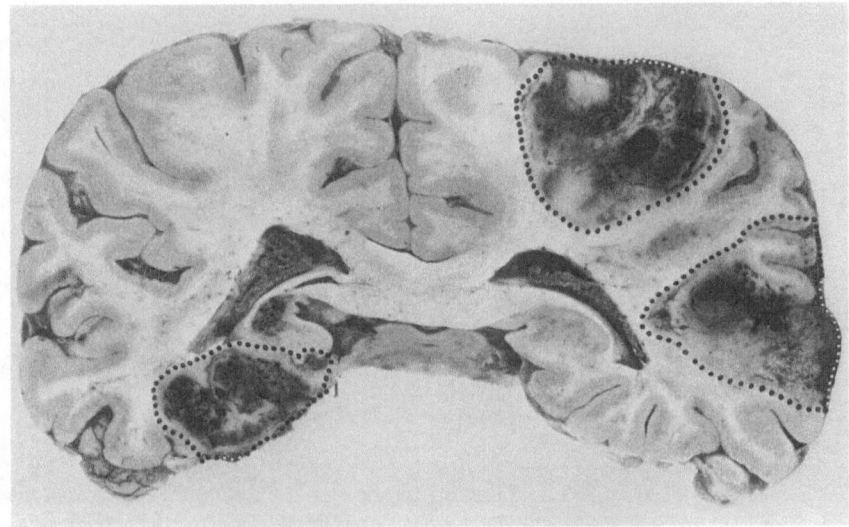

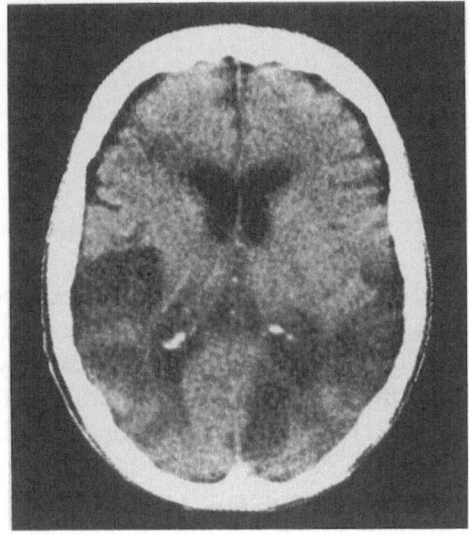

Fig. 28. a Bilateral hemorrhagic infarcts: *left* in supply area of right posterior cerebral artery, and *right* in marginal zones of the left middle cerebral artery. **b** Bilateral infarcts: subtotal *on both sides* in middle cerebral artery as well as subtotal in posterior cerebral artery *on left*

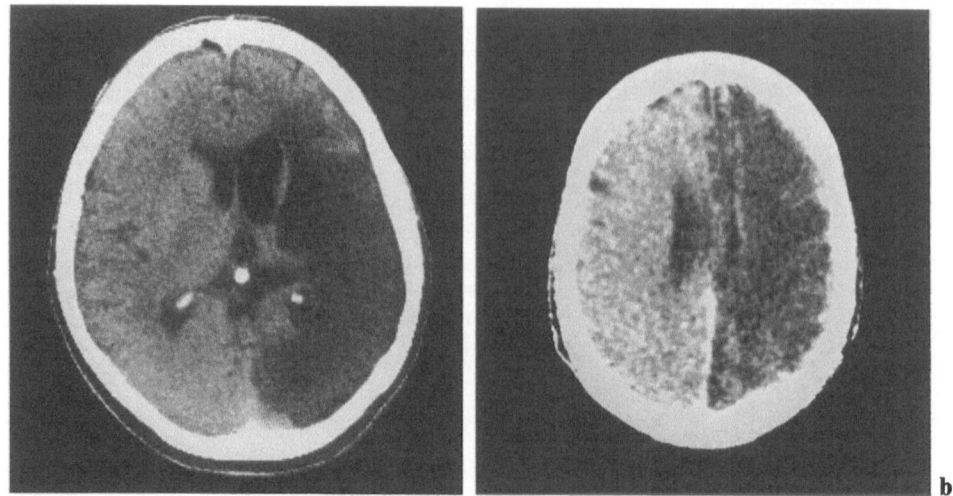

a   b

Fig. 29. a Combined total infarct of middle and posterior cerebral arteries. **b** Complete infarct of one entire hemisphere

1.2 Deep Infarcts in the Area of the Middle Cerebral Artery

Infarcts in the lateral part of the striatopallidum are common. They may be fresh or old, total or spotty, or may be formed according to the principle of the most distant field. In the majority of cases they are hemorrhagic. According to our interpretation, this type of infarct follows in part the Cohnheim principle (by occlusion of the arteries of the basal ganglia). This is always proven when one branch of the lateral striate artery supplies the area around the edge of the lateral ventricle and the infarct includes this zone (see Fig. 30: the borders of this infarct were determined when freshly cut). If, however, a larger portion of the basal ganglia – particularly in the lateral half – is involved and the internal capsule on the other hand only slightly or not at all, or if the infarct extends basally, not only to the edge of the putamen but further into the fronto-orbital convolutions, a watershed/borderline infarction of hemodynamic origin (Figs. 5d and 31a, b) must be assumed. It is located between the territory of the striate arteries and the cortical supply of the middle cerebral artery. On the other hand, partial infarcts, particularly in the distal part of the caudate nucleus and putamen, can with a high degree of certainty be defined as "most distant field" disturbances in the supply area of the striate arteries (Figs. 34a, b and 35a, b).

1.2.1 Infarcts in Putamen and Head of Caudate Nucleus
(Borderline Pattern) (Figs. 30 and 31 a, b)

The occurrence of hemodynamic changes in the border zone between the deep supply of the striate arteries and the superficial circulation of the cortical branches of the middle cerebral artery will influence the pattern and extent of the resulting infarcts. In these cases the internal capsule is widely spared (Fig. 30) because it has only a small number of capillaries and reduced oxygen consumption, which is probably only one-fifth of the putamen and caudate nucleus, which consist of gray matter. Moreover, in these cases the infarcted area usually does not extend into the white substance of the hemispheres, but more basally toward the basal convexity of the brain into the fronto-orbital convolutions (Fig. 31 a).

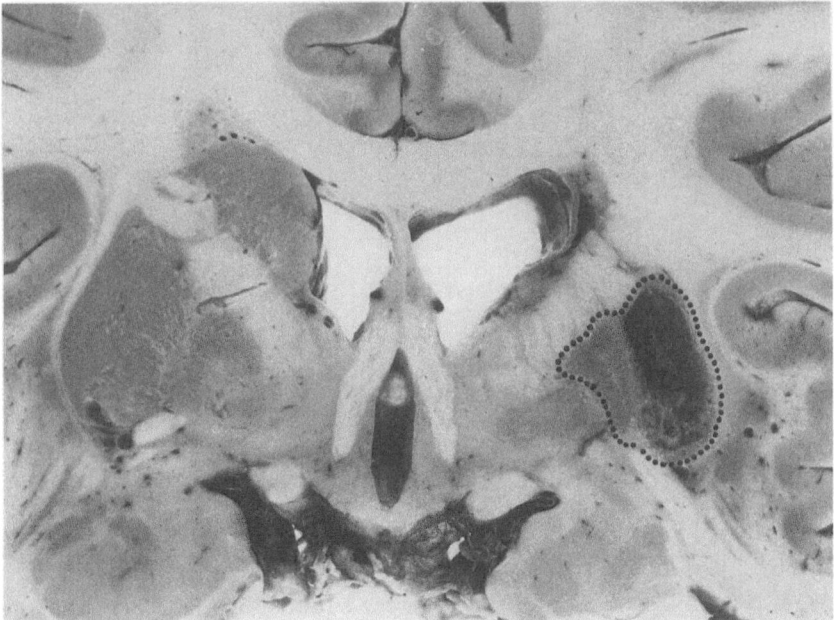

Fig. 30. Complete infarction of medial and lateral striate arteries, now transformed into a cyst (watershed infarct), widely sparing the inner capsule

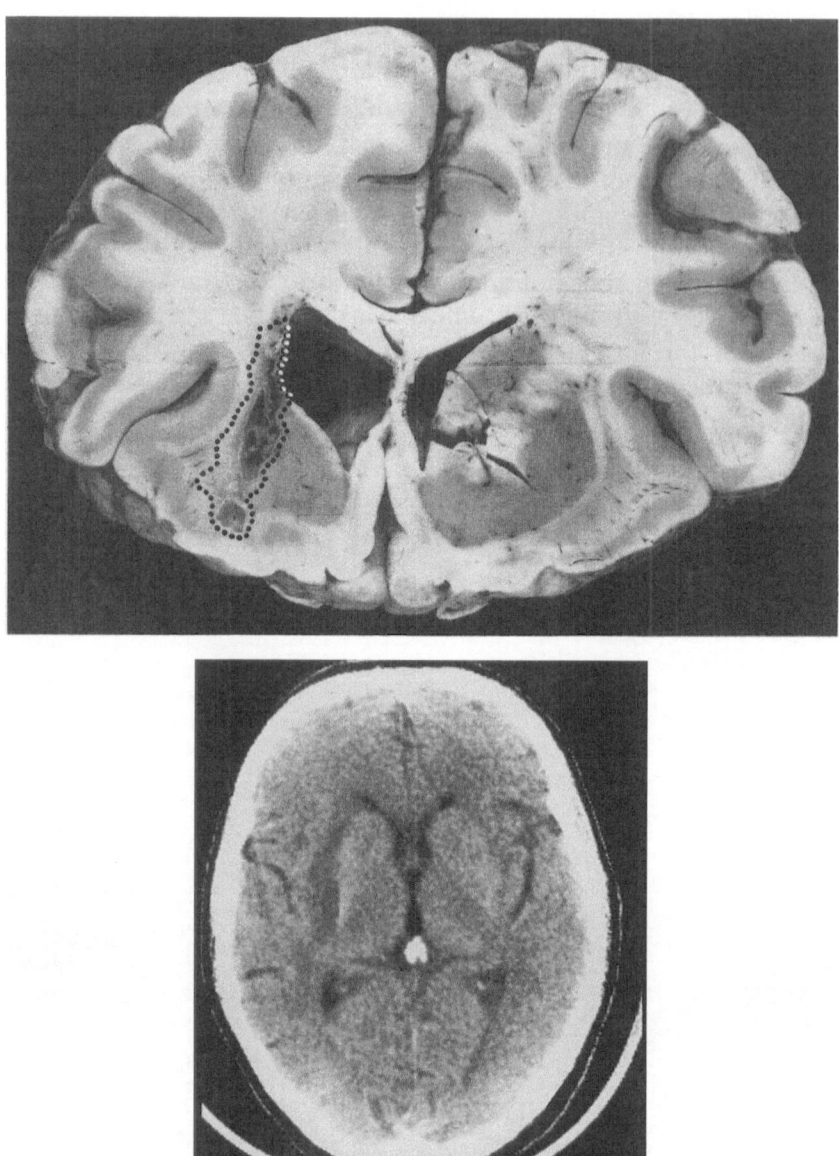

Fig. 31. a Cystic infarct in border zone between left anterior (Heubner's) and middle cerebral arteries. Infarcted area extends up to head of caudate nucleus and down to fronto-orbital convolution (watershed infarct). **b** Partly cystic infarct of putamen with hemorrhagic margin

1.2.2 Total Infarcts of the Striatum
(Fig. 32a, b)

If the middle cerebral artery is occluded precisely at the origin of the medial and lateral striate arteries (Fig. 65 III), a sharply circumscribed, isolated infarct in the striatopallidum may ensue (Figs. 32a, b, 33a, b). The segment supplied by the long central artery (recurrent artery of Heubner) will be spared. Medial parts of the putamen and the head of the caudate nucleus may be preserved as well (Fig. 33a). In some cases the infarct may extend beyond the ventricular border into the white matter, since the lateral striate artery sends a branch into this region, as described by VAN DEN BERGH (1969) (Fig. 33a).

1.2.3 Terminal Infarcts in Putamen and/or Caudate Nucleus
(Most Distant Field) (Figs. 34a, b, 35a, b)

Partial infarcts in the striatum are not rare. Usually the infarcted area involves the distal supply of the striate arteries with location in the head of the caudate nucleus and the dorsal part of the putamen, or only in the caudate nucleus (Fig. 34a, b, 35 a, b). When these infarcts are fresh, they are usually hemorrhagic, but if old they appear as shrunken cystic scars which may produce a deep groove in the ependymal surface of the ventricle (Fig. 35a, b).

1.2.4 Lacunar Infarcts
(Figs. 36–41)

According to FISHER (1969), microinfarcts of 0.5–1.5 cm in size may be called "lacunar" when the affected tissue is transformed into a cyst. FISHER has found them in about 10% of the brains examined by him and the order of frequency was lentiform nucleus → pons → thalamus → caudate nucleus → internal capsule → corona radiata. He did not find any correlation with the well-known forms of vascular insufficiency in the supply area of the internal carotid or with embolism. Moreover, their occurrence was not related to the presence of diabetes mellitus. They occur in children as well (OKUNO et al. 1980), usually as a consequence of trauma. They are found in various parts of the brain, usually in the depths of the white matter in or near the basal ganglia (PULLICINO et al. 1980). MANELFE et al. (1981) attempted to correlate neurologic syndromes with the localization of lacunar infarcts in the internal capsule (Fig. 36a, b).

ZEUMER et al. (1981) have performed a special study of lacunar infarcts. They found them in 11% of their autopsies, 3% being located in the basal

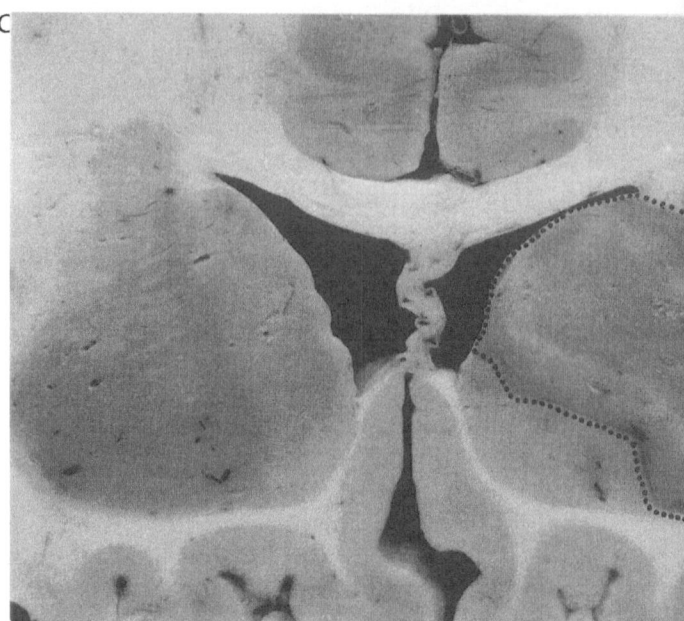

a

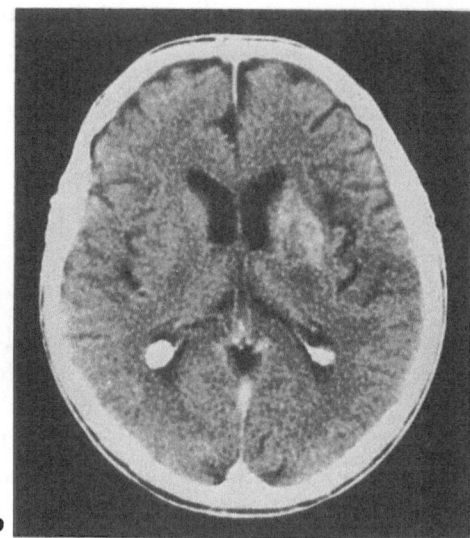

b

Fig. 32. a Hemorrhagic complete infarct in the areas of the medial and lateral striate arteries. **b** Hemorrhagic infarct of lateral striate artery

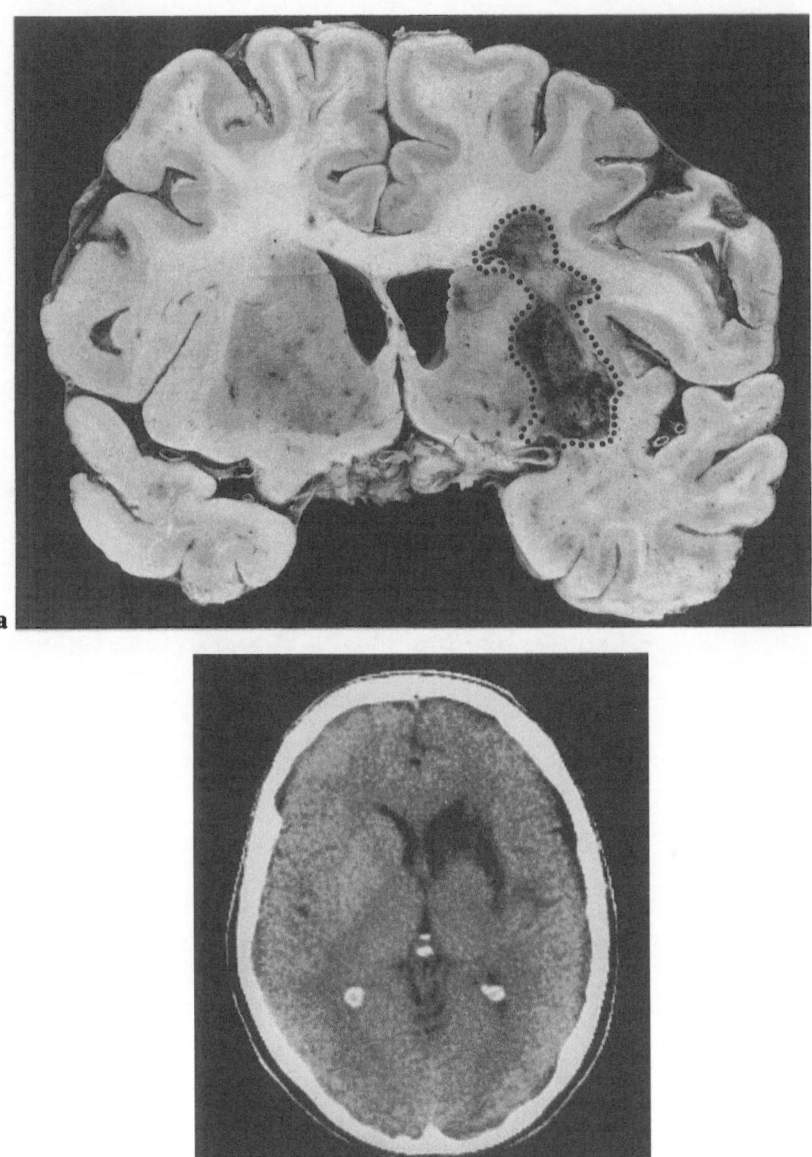

Fig. 33. a Old cystic, formerly hemorrhagic infarct, extending from head of caudate nucleus into semioval center; complete infarct of lateral striate arteries. **b** Old cystic infarct in striatum (complete infarct)

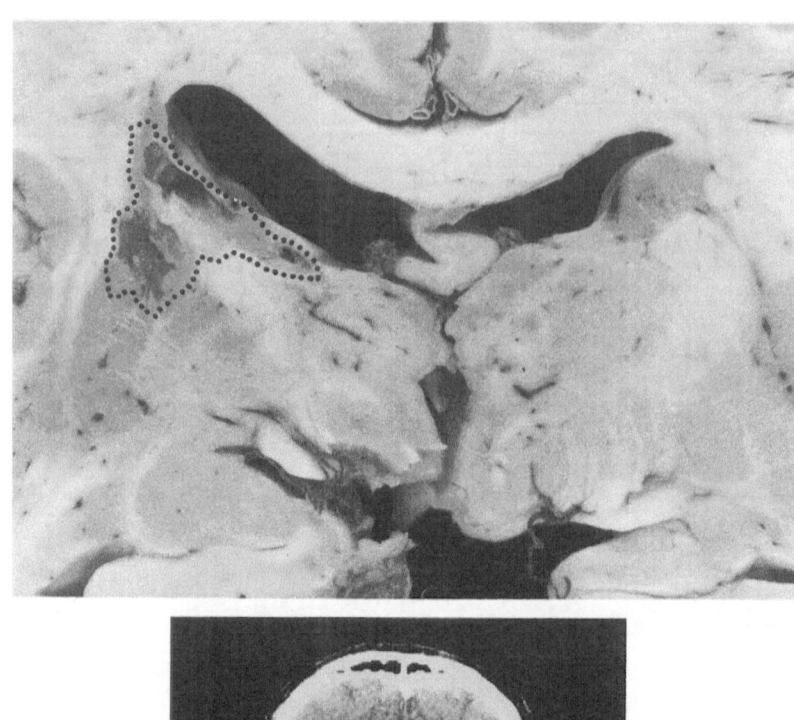

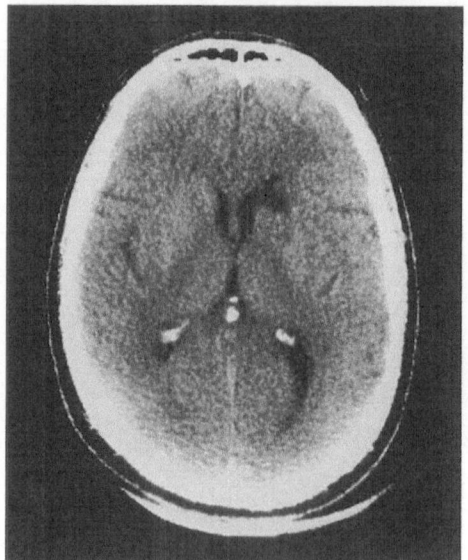

Fig. 34. a Terminal cystic infarct in head of caudate nucleus and upper part of putamen, also involving the internal capsule between the two structures (most distant field infarct). **b** Infarct in the upper third of putamen and head of caudate nucleus (most distant field infarct)

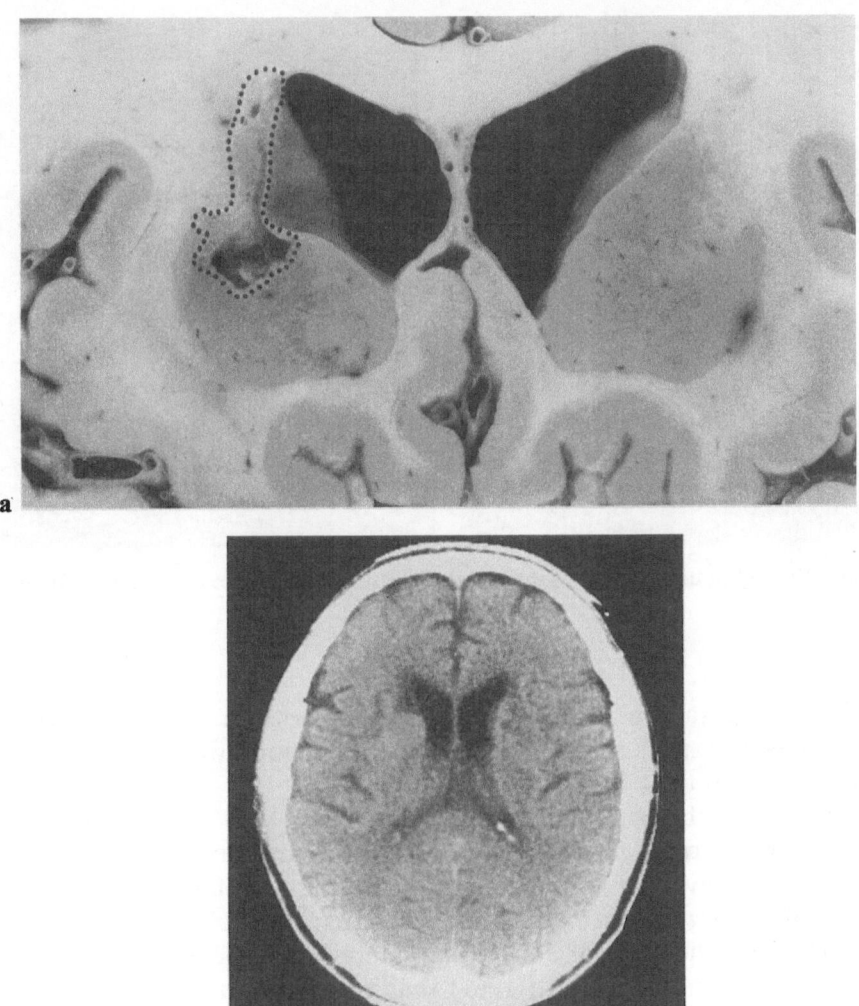

Fig. 35. a Typical deep shrunken groove of an old infarct similar to that in Fig. 34a.
b Typical small infarct at head of caudate nucleus

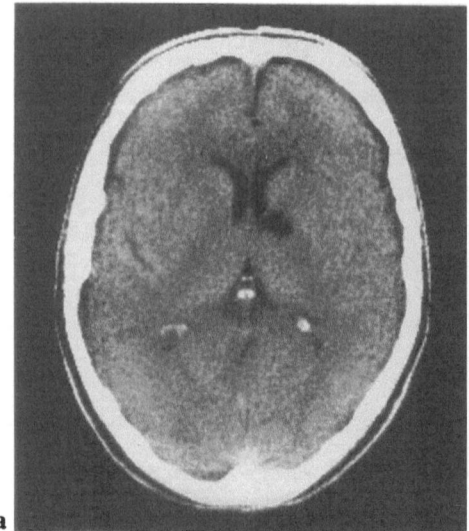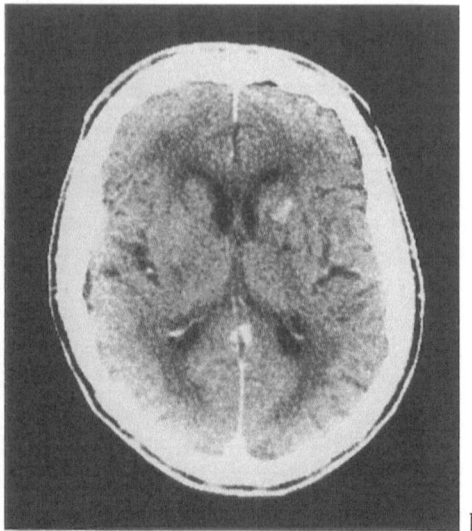

a   b

Fig. 36. a Small (lacunar) infarcts involving the internal capsule. **b** Same type hemorrhagic

ganglia and central white matter. They had a series of 84 cases in which angiography was performed and 109 lacunar lesions were visible in CT scans; in 24 cases these lesions were multiple.

It must be emphasized that the term used by C.M. FISHER (1965, 1969, 1971) for these small cavities predominantly in the putamen and in the pons does not have the same connotation as the original definition of C. and O. VOGT (*état lacunaire*/status lacunaris; see ZÜLCH 1961, 1981, Figs. 107–110). The cysts of *état lacunaire* are hardly demonstrable in CT scans. We have shown (ZÜLCH 1961) that two types of these small cystic infarcts, now termed "lacunar," have a frequent occurrence. Their pathogenesis can readily be explained (ZÜLCH 1981). WODARZ (1980) demonstrated that these particular lacunar infarcts as seen on CT can be pathogenetically explained as we demonstrated earlier (Fig. 8). One of these lacunae is typical of terminal infarction of the striate arteries, whereas the other, situated in the white matter superiorly (Fig. 37a, b) can be explained by the principle of the most distant field, since it occurs in the territory of the perforating branches of the cortical circulation of the middle and anterior cerebral arteries (see Fig. 8).

Two fairly common infarcts of the lacunar type can be found in the proximal (Fig. 38a, b) and terminal territories of the choroidal artery (KLEIHUES 1966) at the outer wall of the ventricular trigone (Fig. 39a, b). The relation of the infarct to this artery was proved by injections of the artery in anatomical specimens.

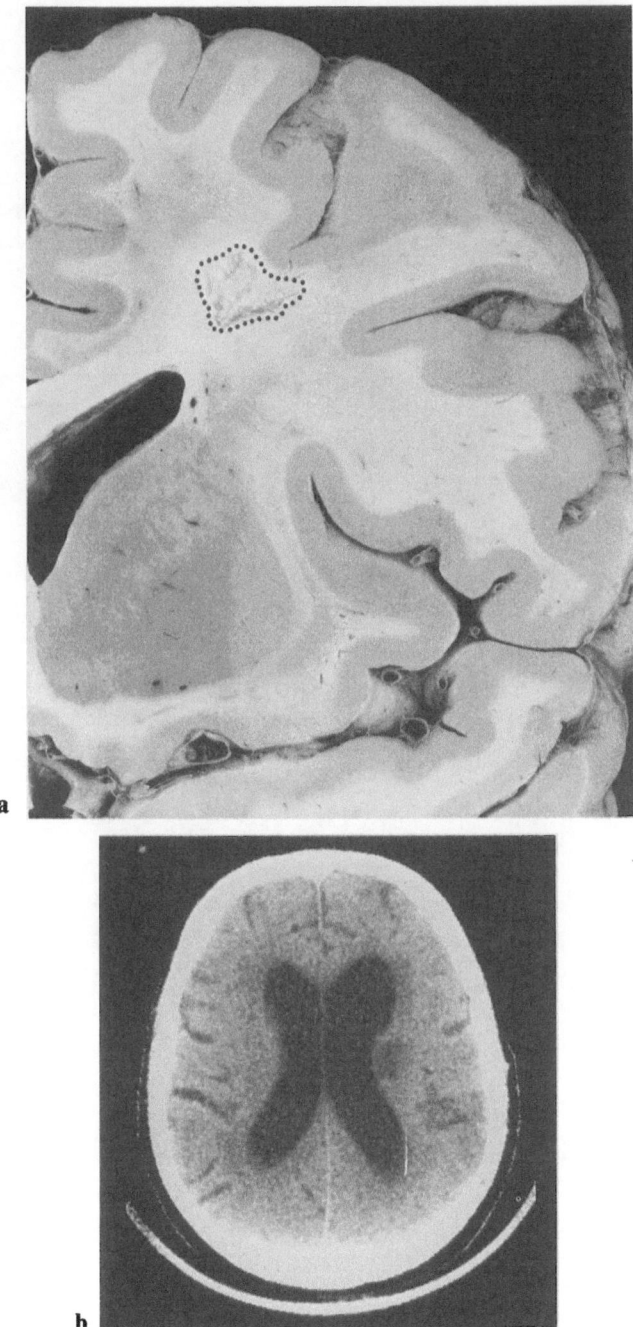

Fig. 37. a Lacunar cystic infarct in semioval center (see Fig. 8). **b** Lacunar infarct in semioval center

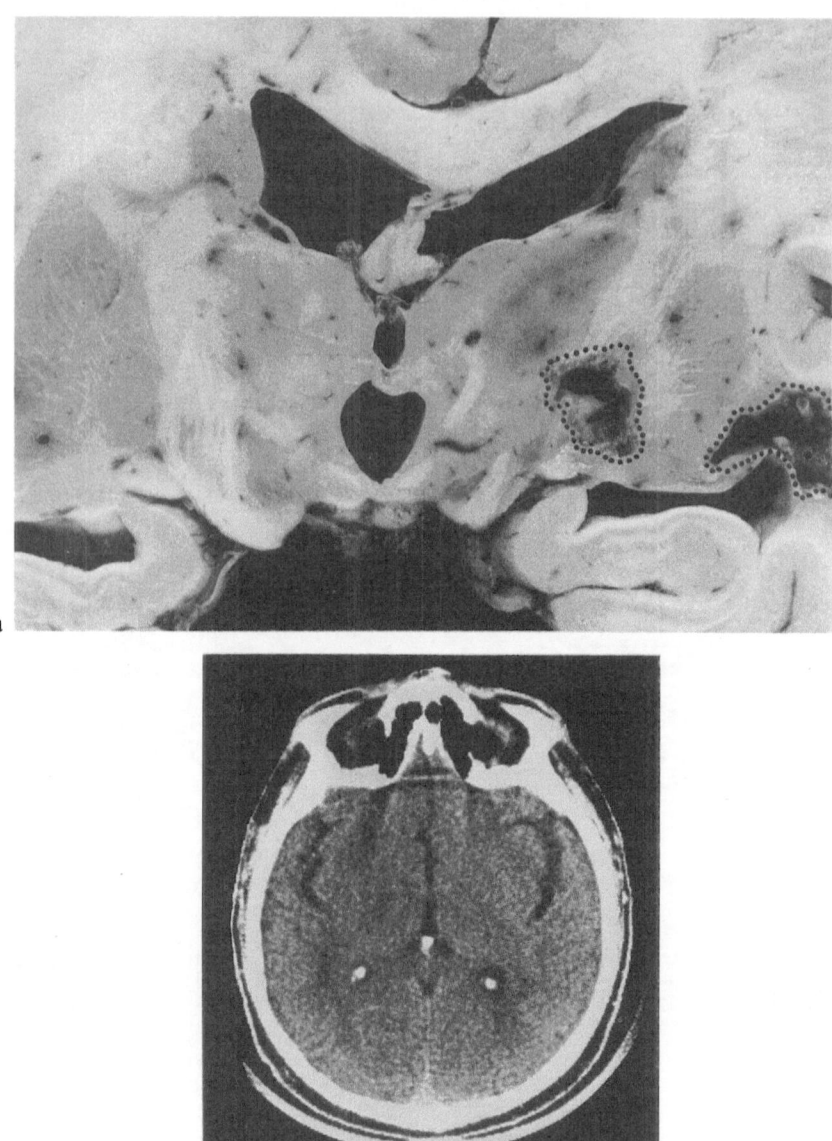

Fig. 38. a Two lacunar cystic infarcts in proximal supply area of anterior choroidal artery. **b** Possible infarct of the medial supply of the anterior choroidal artery

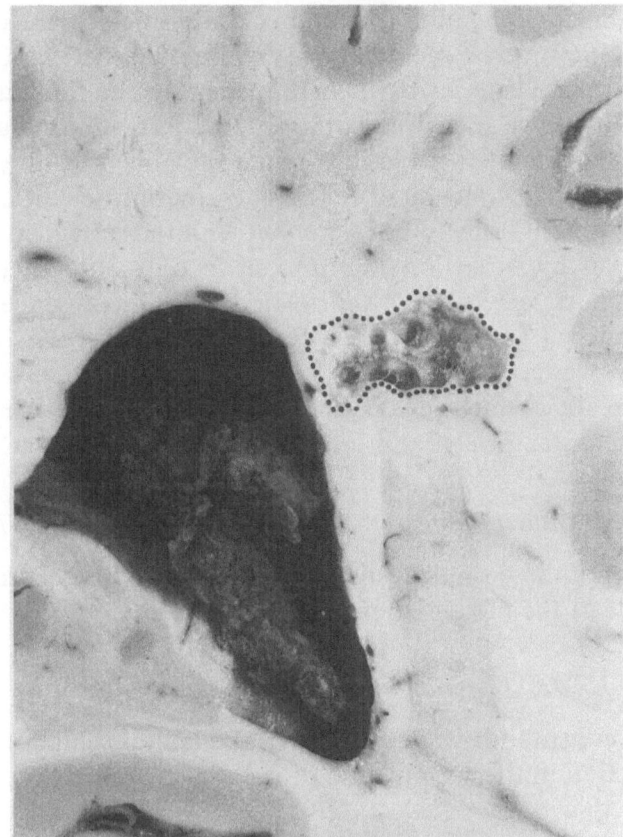

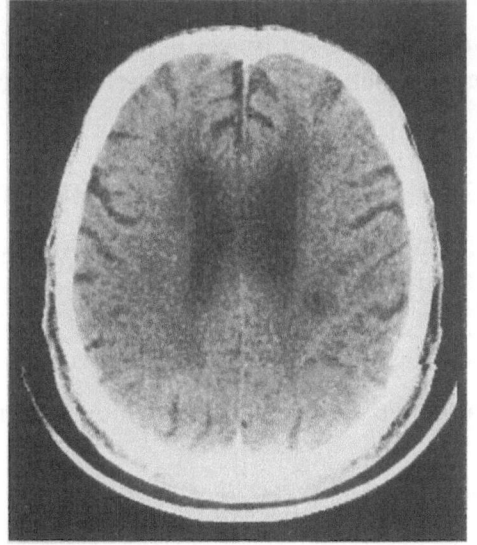

Fig. 39. a Lacunar cystic infarct in terminal supply area of the anterior choroidal artery (lateral wall of trigone). b Large lacunar cystic infarct near wall of trigone (terminal area of anterior choroid artery?)

The typical lacunae in putamen and caudate nucleus are considered by C.M. FISHER (1969) to be secondary to hyalinotic/atheriolosclerotic occlusion of single striate arteries or their branches. In the thalamus and pons, lacunae probably have the same pathogenesis. PULLICINO et al. (1980) emphasized that the size of these lesions remains stable after the first 10 days. If we accept Fisher's concept of hyalinotic/atheriolosclerotic occlusion of striate arteries, we find this to be in conflict with the statement of PULLICINO et al. (1980) that hypertension was present in only 30% of their patients. Hypertension, however, is closely correlated with the presence of hyalinosis in the smaller basal ganglia arteries. In contrast, PULLICINO et al. thought that embolism was a possible pathogenetic mechanism and 21% of their patients had diabetes mellitus. It may very well be that the pathogenesis of lacunae is multifactorial.

1.2.4.1 *Lacunar Infarct in the Semioval Center* (Fig. 37a, b)

This location of these small cystic cavities may also be explained according to the principle of the most distant field (see Fig. 8).

1.2.4.2 *Lacunar Infarct in Thalamus* (Fig. 40a)

This pea-sized, smooth-walled cavity in the lateral thalamus corresponds to microinfarction in the supply area of the thalamogeniculate artery.

1.2.4.3 *Lacunar Infarct in Putamen* (Fig. 40b)

FISHER (1967, 1969) has shown by serial sections that the very common lacunar cysts in the putamen follow hyalinotic/atherosclerotic occlusion of the lateral striate arteries (see above).

1.2.4.4 *Lacunar Infarct in Pons* (Fig. 40c)

These grain-sized, smooth cavities are usually situated in the supply area of the paramedian arteries of the pons.

1.2.4.5 *Lacunar Infarct in Cerebellum*

In the cerebellum, lacunar infarcts of the white matter are rare.

1.2.4.6 *Lacunar Infarcts in the Territory of the Anterior Choroidal Artery* (Fig. 38a, b)

Infarcts in the supply area of the anterior choroidal artery are situated more rostrally in the globus pallidus and at times even extend into a second infarcted zone laterally in the putamen. On the other hand, the caudal

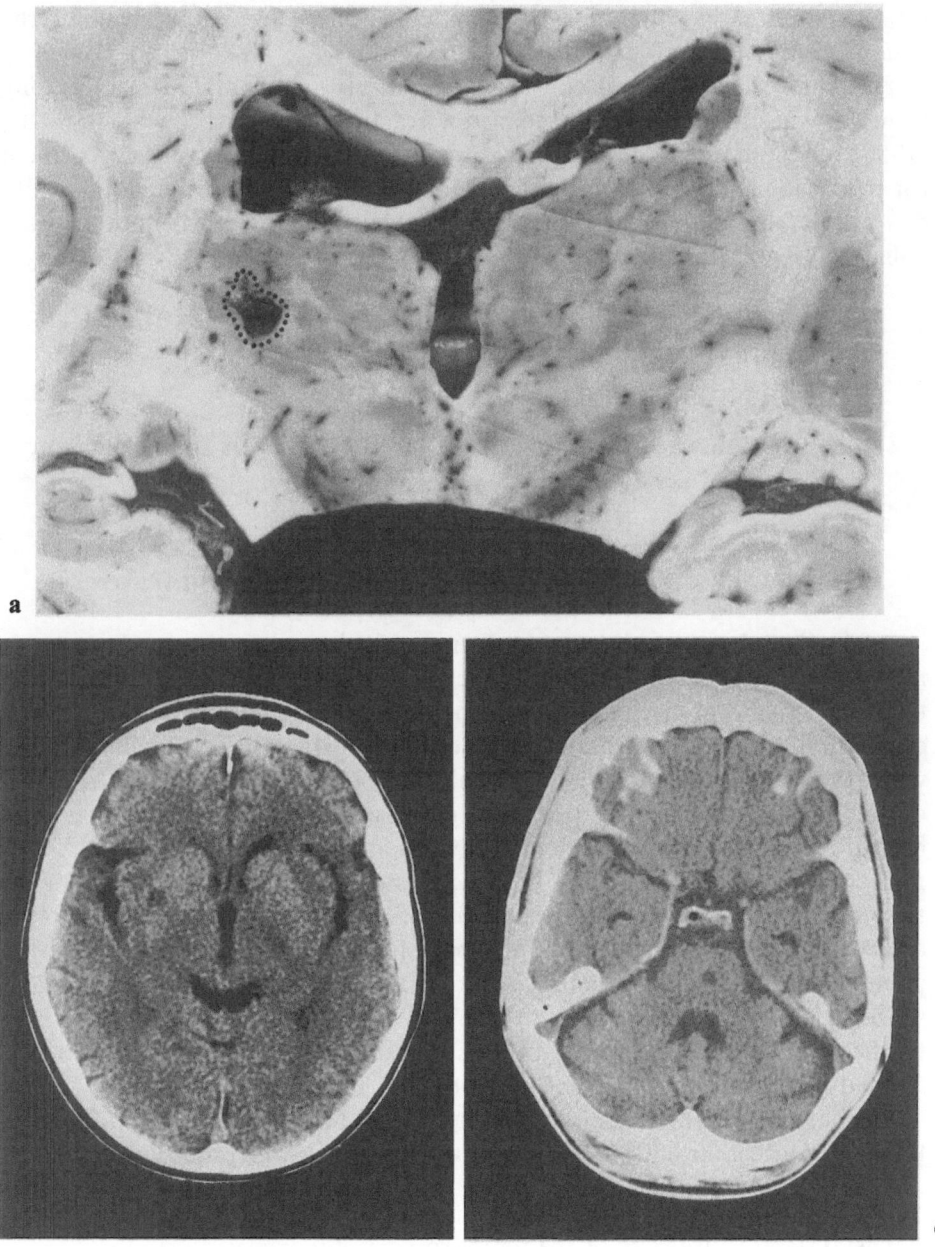

Fig. 40. Lacunar cystic infarct **a** in lateral thalamus, **b** in putamen, **c** in pons

terminal infarct is situated at a distance in the dorsolateral wall of the trigone (Fig. 39a, b) (KLEIHUES 1966).

This curious pattern and course of the anterior choroidal artery has long been known to anatomists. It realized a practical significance when COOPER (1956) recommended the surgical occlusion of this artery as a treatment for parkinsonism. However, the production of an infarct in the globus pallidus was unpredictable because of the variability in the contribution to the collateral circulation by the posterior choroidal artery.

2 The Vertebrobasilar Circulation – Infarcts in the Territory of the Vertebral and Basilar Arteries

2.1 Infarcts in the Territory of the Posterior Cerebral Artery

Infarcts of the posterior cerebral artery territory are extremely variable in their position, extent, and form because, as in the middle cerebral artery territory, collateral circulation may prevent major changes. This collateral circulation functions particularly when the obstruction is proximal, i.e., when there is occlusion of the vertebral artery (Fig. 4). Moreover, the extent of the supply area of the posterior cerebral artery from the uncus and hippocampus to the occipital pole is very long, which provides it with a rich collateral supply through numerous meningeal anastomoses from the two neighboring source arteries, namely the anterior and middle cerebral arteries. If they are functioning, the occipital pole may be adequately supplied by the collaterals, so that a large part of the visual cortex may be spared (KLEIHUES and HIZAWA 1966). A study relating the visual fields to the type of occipital infarction, as demonstrated in CT, has been performed by OSTERTAG and UNSÖLD (1981).

We have tried, therefore, to distinguish seven main types of infarcts of the posterior cerebral artery in accordance with the morphology:

1. Distal (medial) infarcts of the calcarine artery
2. Distal (lateral) infarcts of the temporo-occipital artery
3. Ischemic infarct atrophies of the occipital cortex (rare)
4. Total infarcts of the posterior cerebral artery
5. Bilateral infarcts of the posterior cerebral artery
6. Infarcts in the center of the supply area (in accordance with particular hemodynamic patterns)
8. Spotty infarcts.

One additional fact seems important, namely that when diagnosing ischemic changes in the occipital lobe, one has to consider that this lobe is not usually involved in the cortical atrophy of aging (Fig. 43 a). Therefore, if enlargement of the sulci and atrophy of the convolutions are observed, these changes must be regarded as part of a different pathologic process, mostly of an ischemic nature (see pp. 85, 88 and Fig. 43 b), and not simply atrophy of aging.

Finally, it has to be emphasized that the formation of infarcts in the entire area of the posterior cerebral artery is similar to that in the area of the anterior cerebral artery and may be explained on hemodynamic grounds as well as by the variability of the meningeal anastomoses, as already mentioned. The combination of the posterior cerebral artery infarct with that of the thalamic artery is also quite variable and the combined infarct is only visible in a small proportion of cases. Curiously enough, there may also be a medial infarct in the distal part of the occipital lobe combined with a smaller infarct in the territory of the thalamogeniculate artery without any communication between the two or other spotty locations. We did not, however, find embolism to be a likely explanation (see Fig. 4).

2.1.1 Infarcts of the Calcarine Artery (Medial Occipital Infarct)
(Fig. 41 a, b)

As we have emphasized above, in the majority of cases it is not the entire supply area (Fig. 41 a, b) of the posterior cerebral artery which is involved when the artery is occluded. Usually, only single large branches are affected: for example, the medial branch, the calcarine artery, or only the most distal branch supplying the occipital pole. In these cases the entire medial surface of the occipital lobe is totally or spotty infarcted (Fig. 41 a). This is a type of infarct commonly observed in CT (Fig. 41 b). Defects in the area of the calcarine artery are different in their location and extent. The action of the neighboring meningeal anastomoses may be variable. They contribute by collateral circulation to a shrinking of the infarcted area. KLEIHUES and HIZAWA (1966) clearly demonstrated this concept in a schematic drawing of the size and location of the infarcted areas (onion-like pattern).

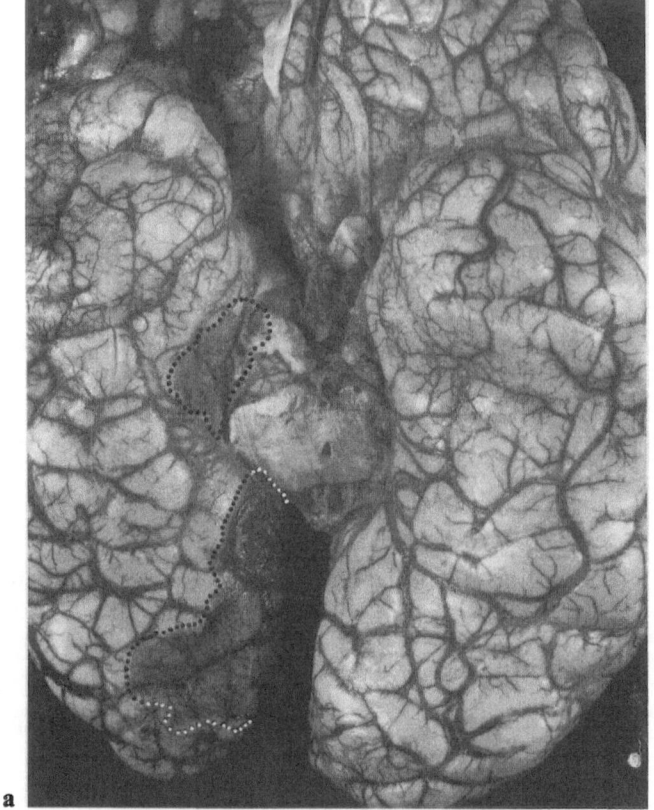

a

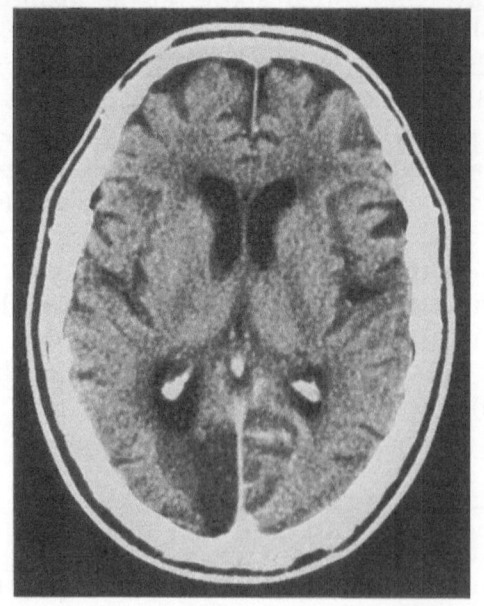

b

2.1.2 Infarcts of the Occipitotemporal Artery (Lateral Occipital Infarct)
(Fig. 42a, b)

The infarct of the occipitotemporal artery, e.g., lateral part of the occipital lobe, is less common than that of the calcarine artery. Neither the clinical picture nor the very precise investigation of KLEIHUES and HIZAWA (1966) clarifies the reason for the occurrence of either of these two types of infarcts.

2.1.3 Cortical Infarcts Within the Area of the Posterior Cerebral Artery
(Fig. 43a, b)

In a few cases, cerebrovascular insufficiency within the posterior cerebral artery territory occurs, leading to a more generalized cortical atrophy (a rare event among the ischemic lesions of the occipital lobe). It may be that this is due to partial occlusion of the artery or, as we have seen in one of our cases, a probable embolism. We have always emphasized that this part is never involved in cortical atrophy of the aged (see also pp. 85, 88).

2.1.4 Total Infarct of the Posterior Cerebral Artery
(Figs. 44a, b and 45a, b)

With this total infarct, the entire supply area of the posterior cerebral artery may be involved, although not always completely. The most common area affected comprises the uncus and medial part of the temporal lobe, the lateral part of the convexity just above the base of the brain, the occipital pole, the medial part of the occipital lobe including the calcarine convolution, and the neighboring inferior temporal and occipitotemporal gyri. This type of infarct is not infrequently hemorrhagic. Subtotal infarcts usually spare the process in the transverse direction, whereas longitudinal infarction from the occipital pole to the uncus and hippocampus along their total length is more common. This is readily understood when one considers that the lateral edges of this territory are more satisfactorily supplied by meningeal anastomoses from the middle cerebral artery.

Fig. 41. a Incomplete hemorrhagic infarct in irrigation area of right posterior cerebral artery (predominantly medial infarct). **b** Infarct of distal posterior cerebral artery (predominantly in area of calcarine artery; medial infarct)

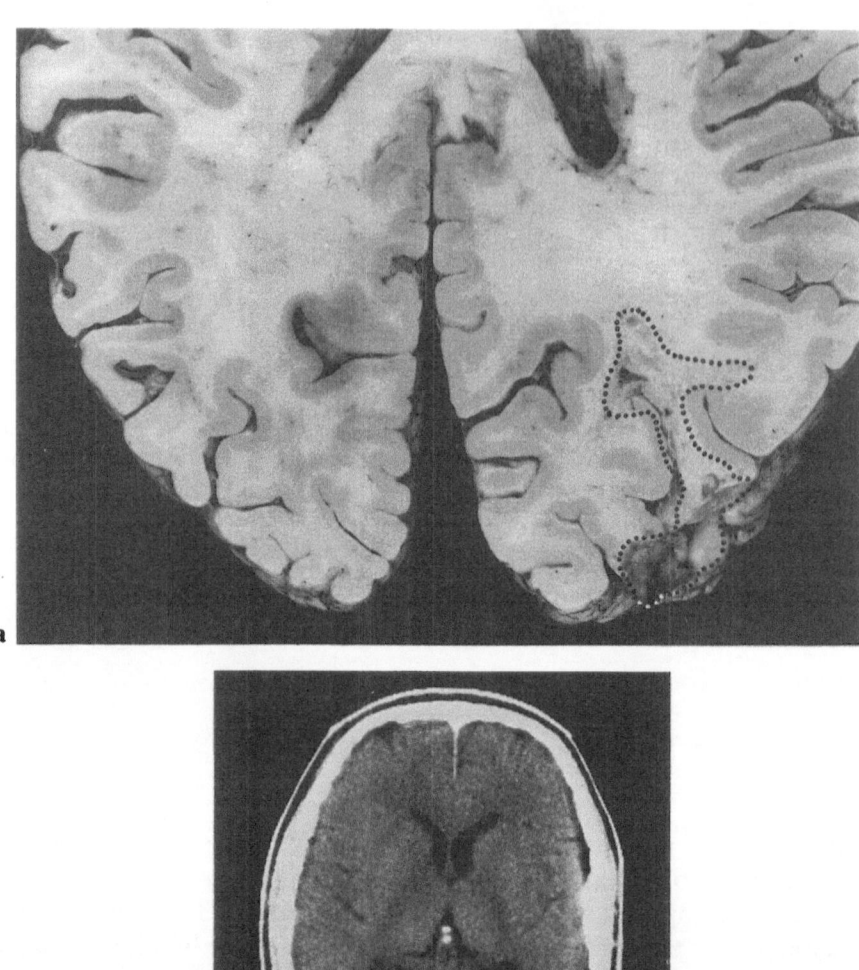

Fig. 42. a Predominantly lateral infarct of posterior cerebral artery. **b** Predominantly laterally situated infarct of posterior cerebral artery (occipitotemporal artery)

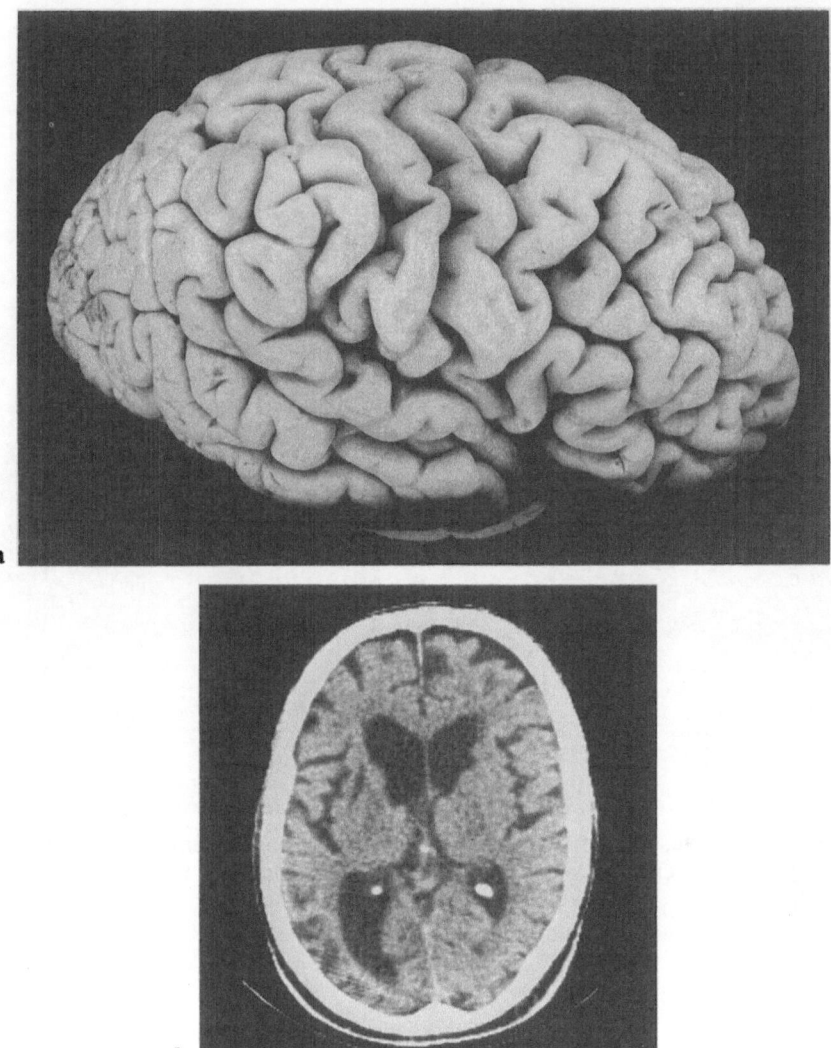

Fig. 43. a Brain with marked atrophy exceeding highest normal degree for age. Sparing of fissures of occipital lobe is easily recognized. **b** Ischemic atrophy of right occipital cortex (after embolism). Enlarged brain sulci and lateral ventricle (trigone/occipital horn)

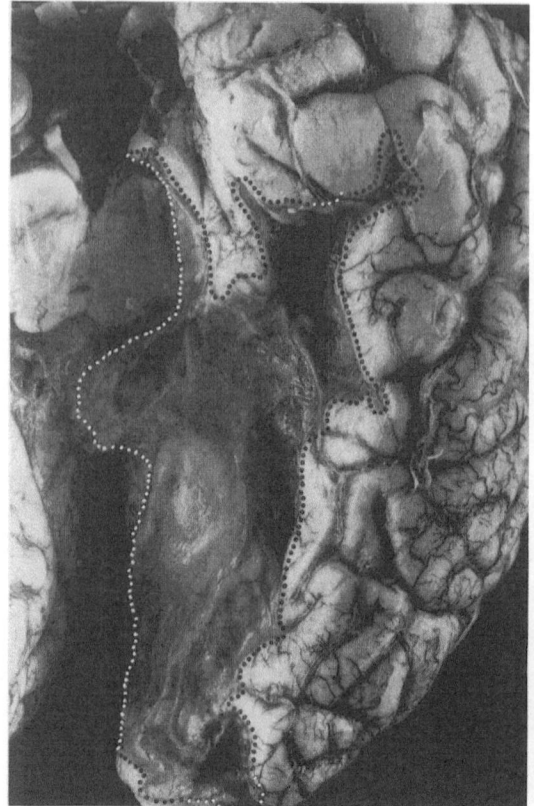
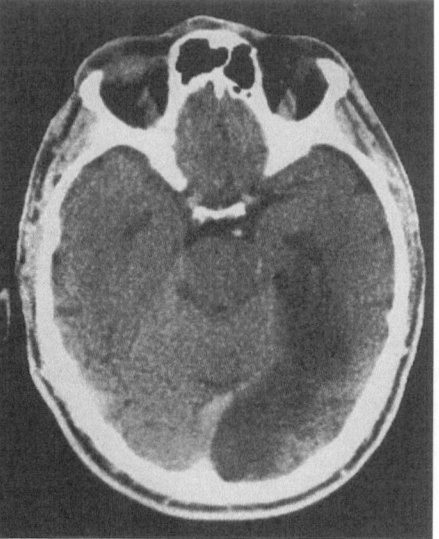

a

b

Fig. 44. a Extensive, almost complete, cystic and formerly hemorrhagic infarct in area of posterior cerebral artery (predominantly medial). **b** Complete infarct of posterior cerebral artery

2.1.5 Bilateral Infarcts of the Posterior Cerebral Arteries
(Fig. 45a, b)

As opposed to infarcts within the middle cerebral artery, bilateral infarcts within the supply area of the posterior cerebral artery are not uncommon; however, they may not be symmetrical. This bilateral occurrence is explained by the supply of both posterior cerebral arteries from a single artery, namely the basilar artery in four-fifths of the cases. It will be extremely rare for this type of infarct to be total on both sides. On the contrary, distal parts of the supply areas are preferred. Hence complete blindness may occur as a consequence of bilateral involvement of the calcarine area.

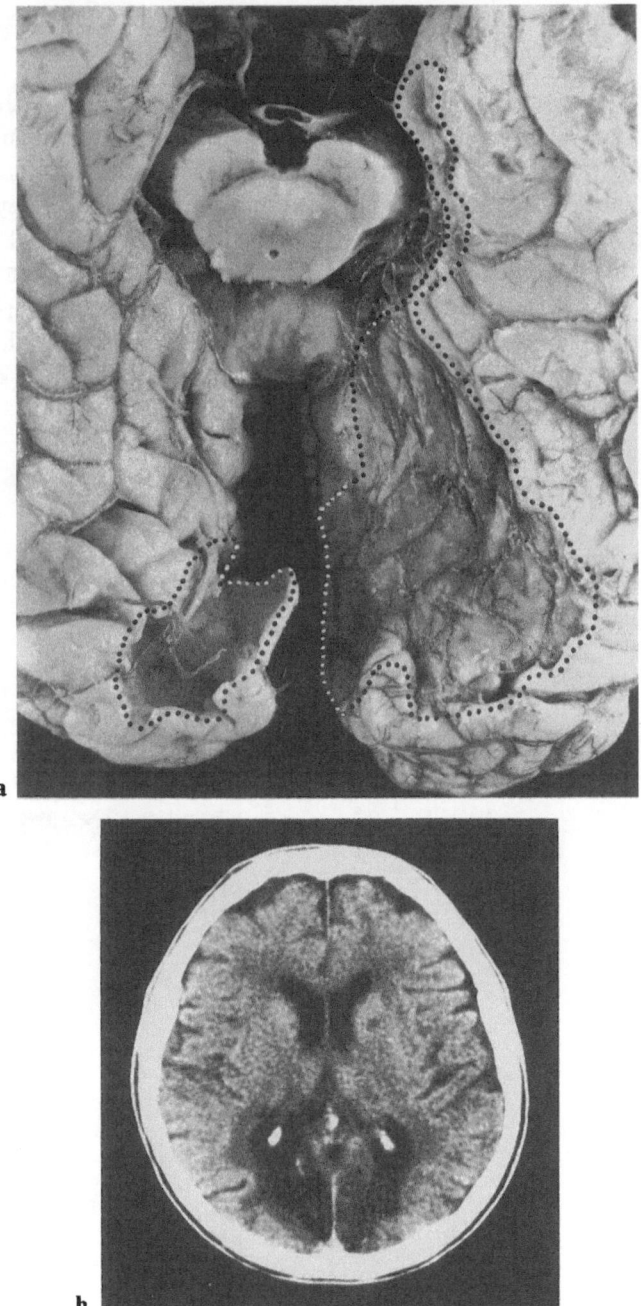

Fig. 45. a Bilateral complete cystic infarcts in irrigation area of both posterior cerebral arteries. **b** Bilateral infarcts of posterior cerebral arteries

2.1.6 Infarcts in the Center of the Territory of the Posterior Cerebral Artery
(Fig. 46a, b)

Infarcts are common in the center of the supply area of the posterior cerebral arteries (see p. 11). They follow a vertebrobasilar insufficiency if one of the posterior cerebral arteries is stenosed at the same time, e.g., when general and local factors are hemodynamic operative. They also occur as a consequence of either persistent or intermittent tentorial herniation. This type of infarct was described as early as 1938 by MOORE and STERN and in 1939 by RIESSNER and ZÜLCH, who provided excellent pictures and made extensive studies regarding this phenomenon (ZÜLCH et al. 1974). The infarcts are situated slightly below the calcarine fissure (ZÜLCH and KLEIHUES 1967, Figs. 10 and 11).

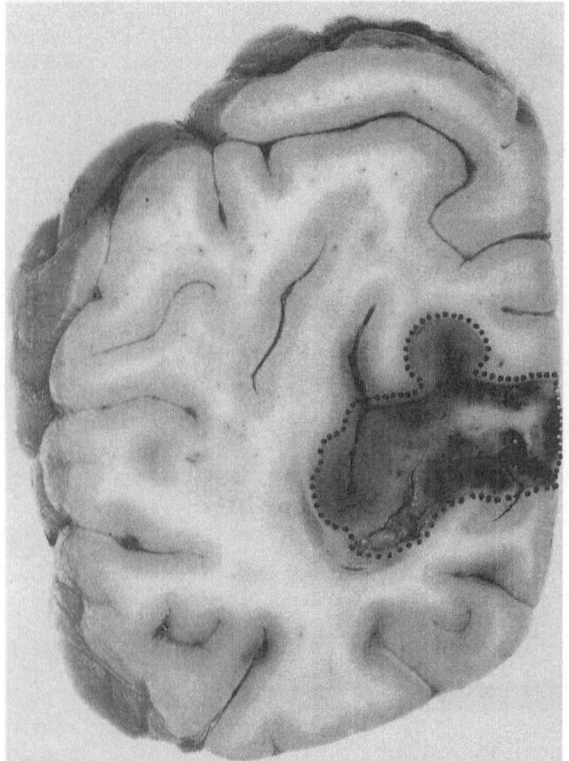
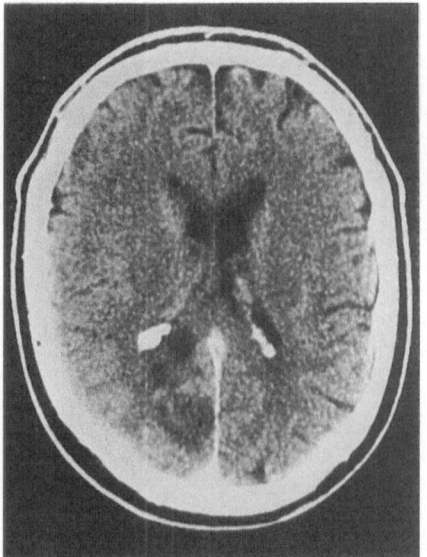

a   b

Fig. 46. a Relatively fresh hemorrhagic infarct in the center of the supply area of posterior cerebral artery. **b** Typical infarct in center of supply area of right posterior cerebral artery

2.2 Infarcts in Thalamus (Thalamogeniculate and Thalamoperforate Arteries) (Fig. 47 a–c)

Two types of infarcts are encountered in the thalamus which correspond in their location to the territories of supply of the thalamoperforate and thalamogeniculate arteries. They are, in the majority, of a hemorrhagic nature and only rarely is the entire supply area of both arteries compromised. More often they occur in isolation, and only in occasional cases do we see a really total infarction of the posterior cerebral artery, including the thalamus.

The infarcts stemming from the perforating arteries have a medial location. In contrast, the more distally originating thalamogeniculate arteries, when occluded, produce an infarct in the lateral part of the thalamus. Typically, the geniculate body is infarcted.

2.3 Infarcts in Cerebellum
(Figs. 48 a, b–51 a, b)

Cerebellar infarcts are very rarely total. Commonly, only circumscribed small infarcts occur either on the dorsal or the ventral surface, depending on which of the two source arteries is involved, the superior or anterior inferior cerebellar artery. These cerebellar infarcts generally do not correspond to the total supply area but are localized in the center of the irrigating area. Apparently, meningeal anastomoses can operate very effectively in the cerebellum. Watershed infarcts are also observed. They originate at the lateral margins of the cerebellar hemispheres and presumably have a hemodynamic origin. By the time pathologists see these cerebellar infarcts they are already old, since they are usually relatively small and seldom endanger the life of the patient.

2.3.1 Dorsal Cerebellar Infarct (Superior Cerebellar Artery)
(Fig. 48 a, b)

The dorsal cerebellar infarct is localized within the center of the supply area and only rarely occurs as a terminal infarct of the superior cerebellar artery. The extent of the compromised area is usually reduced by the numerous meningeal anastomoses of the neighborhood.

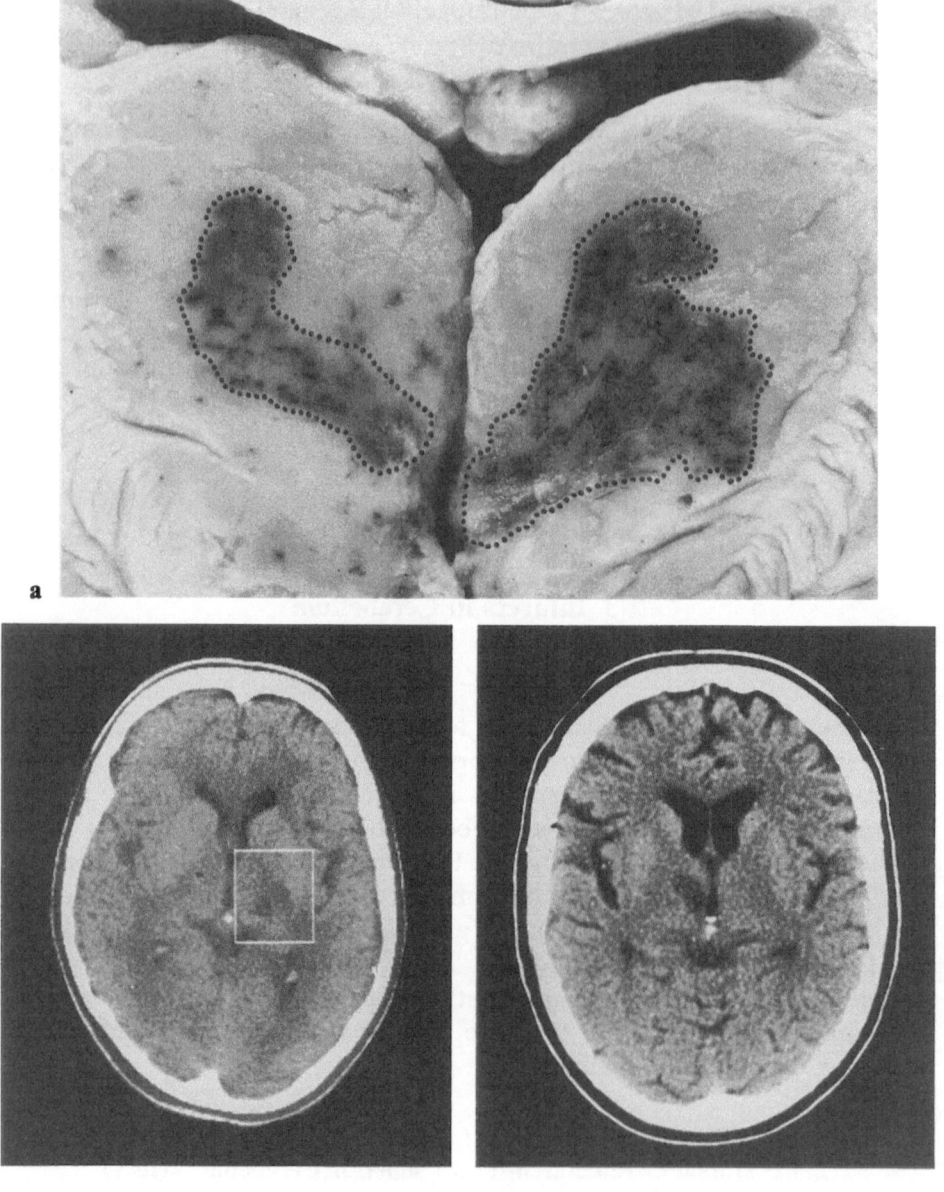

Fig. 47. a Bilateral, hemorrhagic, partial infarcts in the area of the thalamoperforate artery. **b** Infarct in dorsolateral thalamus (thalamogeniculate artery). **c** Infarct in medial thalamus

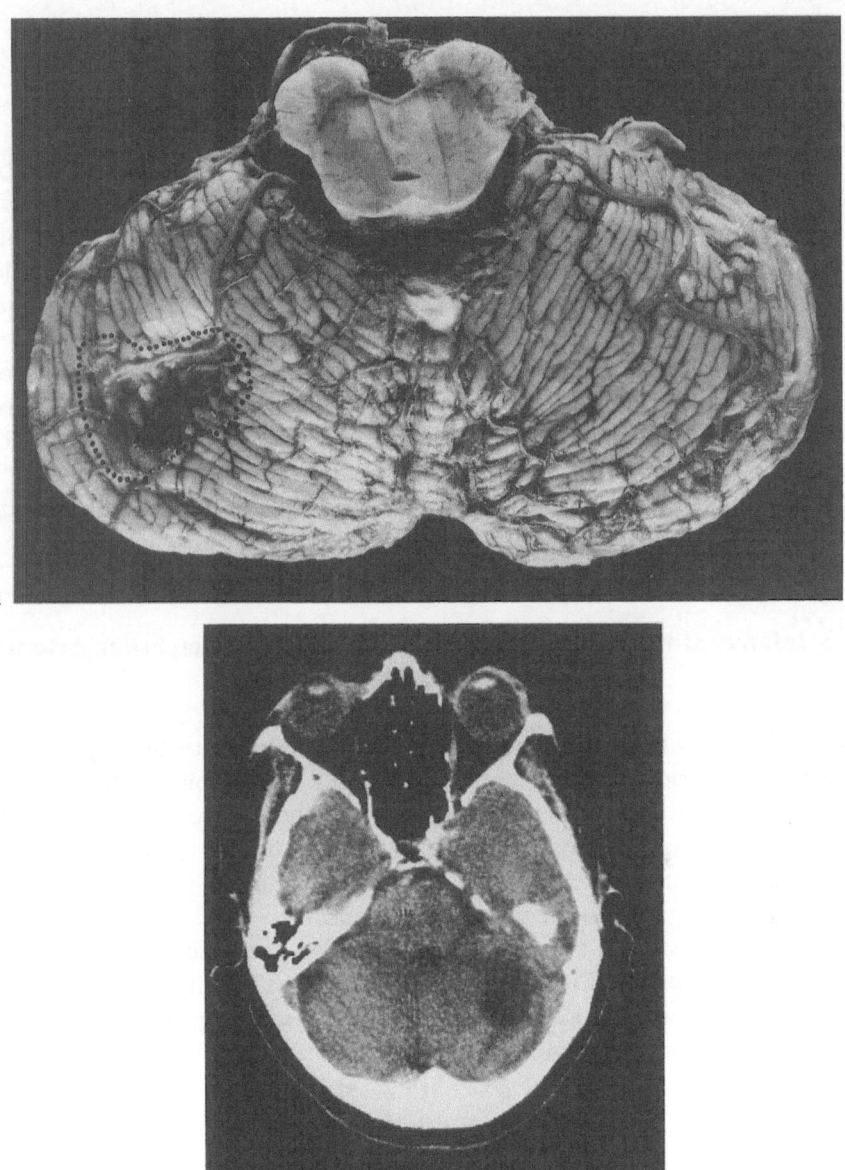

Fig. 48. a Deeply grooved, small, crater-like dorsal cerebellar infarct. **b** Dorsal cerebellar infarct in supply area of superior cerebellar artery

2.3.2 Ventral Cerebellar Infarcts (Anterior Inferior Cerebellar Artery)
(Figs. 49 a, b and 50 a, b)

The ventral infarct of the cerebellum either covers the area near the midline, which is a major part of the supply area of the anterior inferior cerebellar artery, or it may be located more laterally, in which case it is smaller.

It is rare for an infarct to be situated on the ventral surface in the supply area of the posterior inferior cerebellar artery (Wallenberg artery) unless it is combined with corresponding small infarcts in the medulla oblongata (the dorsolateral infarct of the medulla oblongata) (Fig. 55).

The posterior inferior cerebellar artery may present itself either as one branch from the basilar artery or as two smaller branches, of which one supplies the cerebellar area and the other runs directly to the medulla oblongata.

Occasionally, cerebellar infarcts are bilateral and are then usually situated in analogous areas (Fig. 50 b).

2.3.3 Infarcts at the Watersheds (Border Zone) of the Cerebellar Arteries
(Fig. 51 a, b)

Some of the cerebellar infarcts cannot be correlated with the supply areas of the main arteries. They are, however, understandable if the principle of endangering the watersheds is applied. In these cases one sees at the borderline between superior cerebellar arteries and the posterior inferior or anterior inferior cerebellar arteries deeply shrunken infarcted grooves, often suggesting a previous hemorrhagic character.

Small infarcts occur on the cerebellar ventral or dorsal surfaces as terminal lesions due to occlusion of branches of the arteries. They are not uncommon, although they are usually so small that they are not diagnosed in CT scans because of the potential artifacts encountered in this region. One can demonstrate them with certainty only with thin slices.

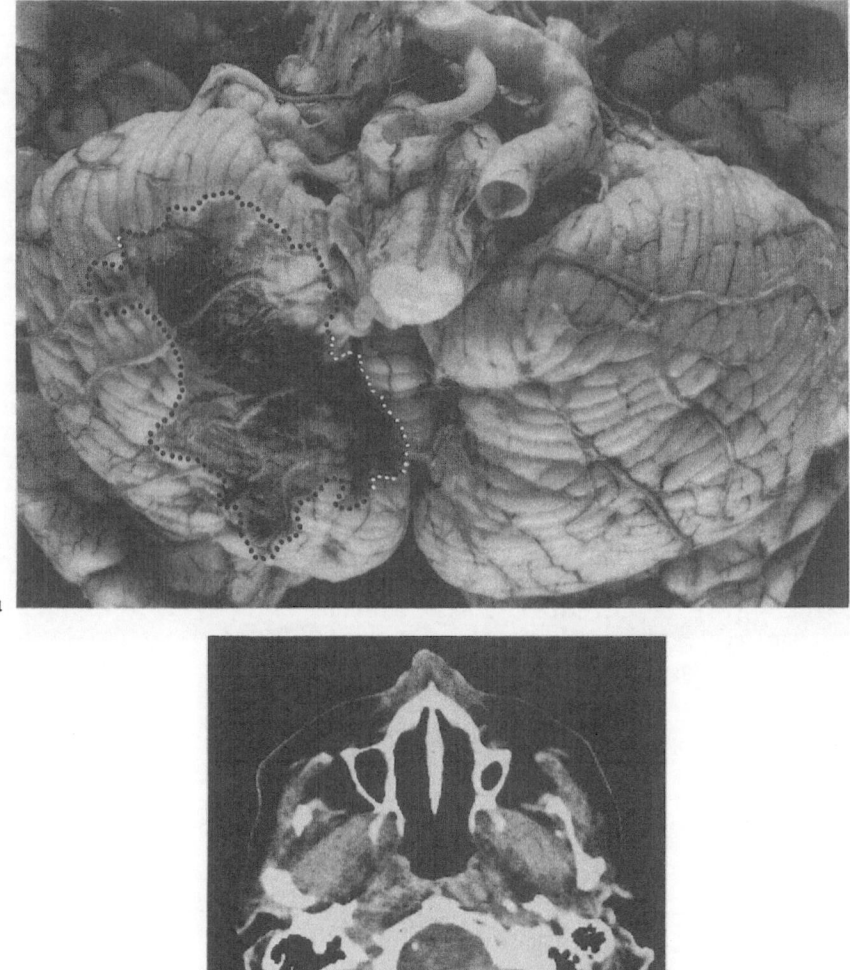

Fig. 49. a Medium-sized, deeply grooved ventral infarct of anterior inferior cerebellar artery. **b** Ventral cerebellar infarct of anterior inferior cerebellar artery

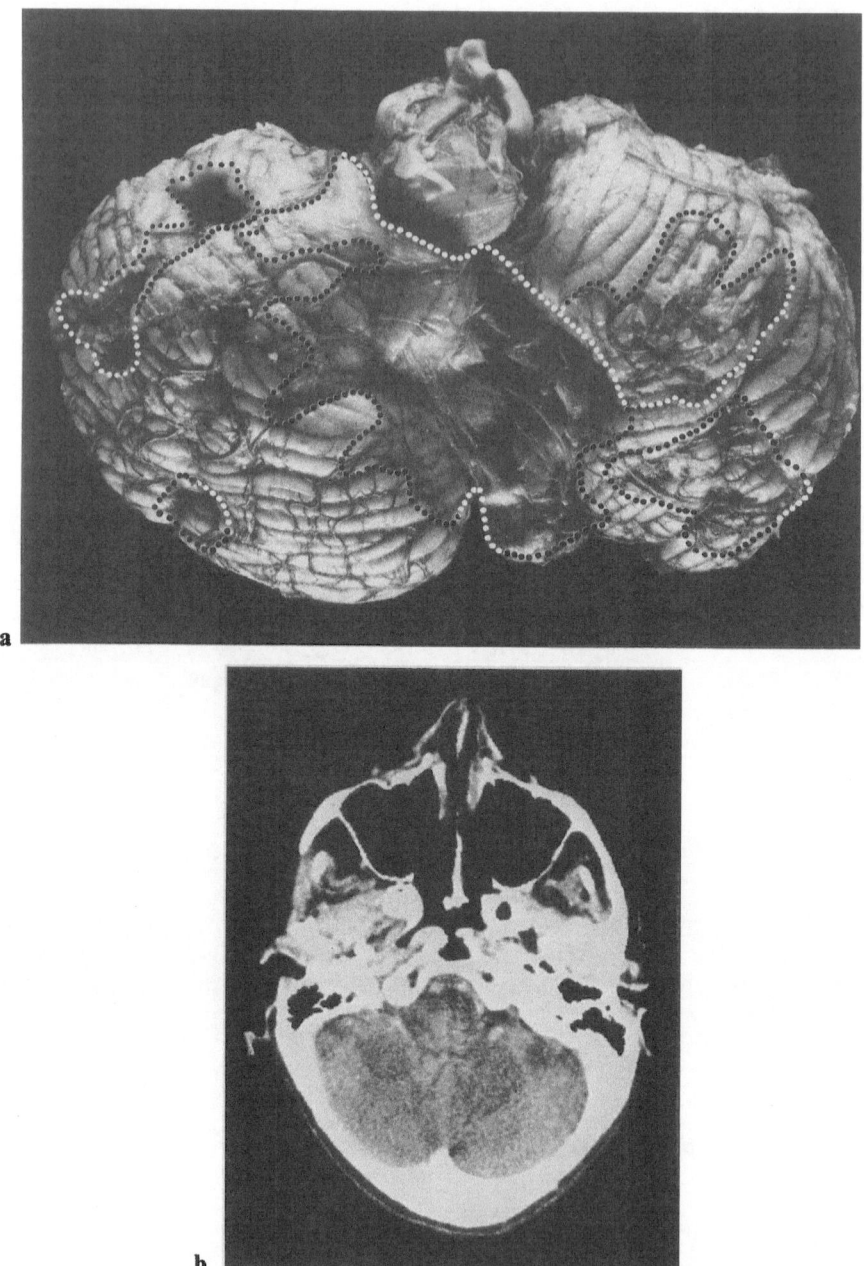

Fig. 50. a Superficial system of grooved cerebellar infarcts in both hemispheres of cerebellum (ventral). **b** Superficial ventral infarcts of cerebellum

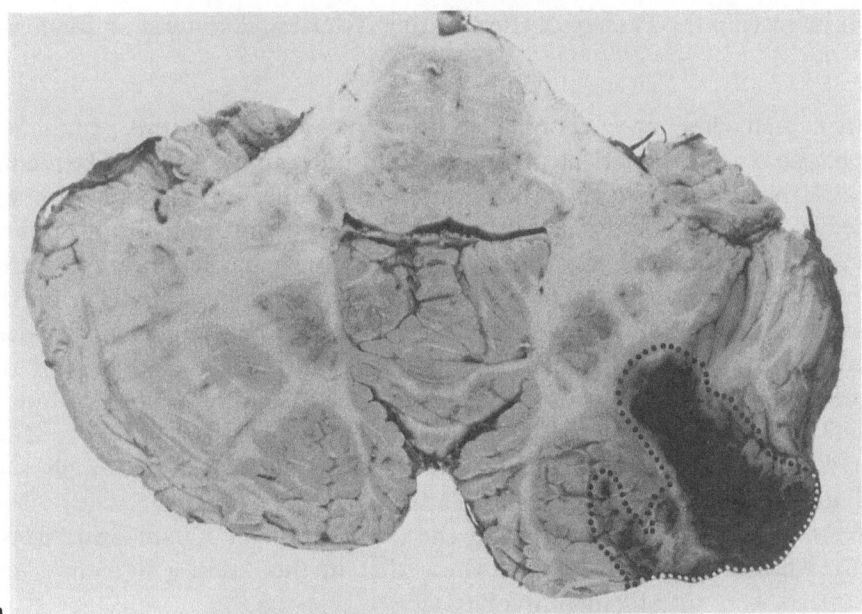

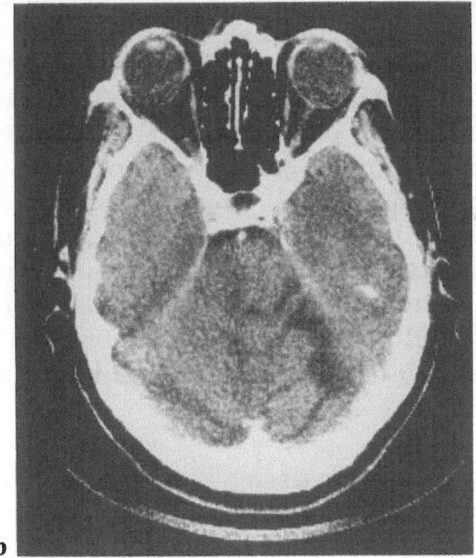

Fig. 51. a Hemorrhagic infarct in watershed area between superior and anterior inferior cerebellar arteries. **b** Infarct in watershed area between superior and anterior inferior cerebellar arteries

2.3.4 Infarcts in the Pedunculi (Perforating Arteries, Unilateral or Bilateral) (Fig. 52a, b)

When analyzing mesencephalic infarcts, particularly in the peduncular region, one must consider the arrangement of the source arteries. The medial parts of the pedunculi are directly supplied by the paramedian branches of the basilar artery, or else from proximal segments of the posterior cerebral artery. The dorsolateral and tectal regions, on the other hand, are irrigated by the superior cerebellar artery, which artery also stems directly from the basilar artery. There may be excellent collateral circulation from the meningeal anastomoses of the neighborhood, so that the dorsal parts of the mesencephalon are more protected from ischemia than the ventral peduncular parts. This will explain the almost invariable integrity of the suprapeduncular tectal parts of the mesencephalon seen in our cases, although very small grain-like lacunae may be visible (Fig. 52a).

We emphasize this in contrast to the observation of KUBIK and ADAMS (1946), who in their basic article show that in their series tegmental and tectal parts were usually also involved.

Due to the different vascular supply of the pedunculi, those medial parts which are supplied by the perforating branches of the basilar artery can be infarcted, while lateral parts still obtain blood supply through meningeal anastomoses from the posterior cerebral artery. This can occur when the occluding thrombus has not propagated from the basilar artery into the two posterior cerebral arteries. Moreover, it has to be kept in mind that in 20% of cases the "embryonal" type of posterior cerebral artery will be present, with which there is an origin of the posterior cerebral artery directly from the internal carotid artery. In such cases, the posterior cerebral artery territory will be sufficiently supplied to protect it from infarction.

The frequent bilateral infarction of the pedunculi is explained by the source of the supply from one artery, namely the basilar artery.

2.3.5 Infarcts of Pons (Paramedian Pontine Artery, Short and Long Circumflex Arteries) (Figs. 53a–c and 54a, b)

There are two markedly different infarcts in the pons, those of the medial (paramedian) artery (Fig. 53a–c) and the lateral (long circumflex) artery and, in the territory between these, the rather rare intermediate infarcts (short circumflex artery). At autopsy these infarcts often appear in the form of a long deep cystic cavity. They can be survived for a long time.

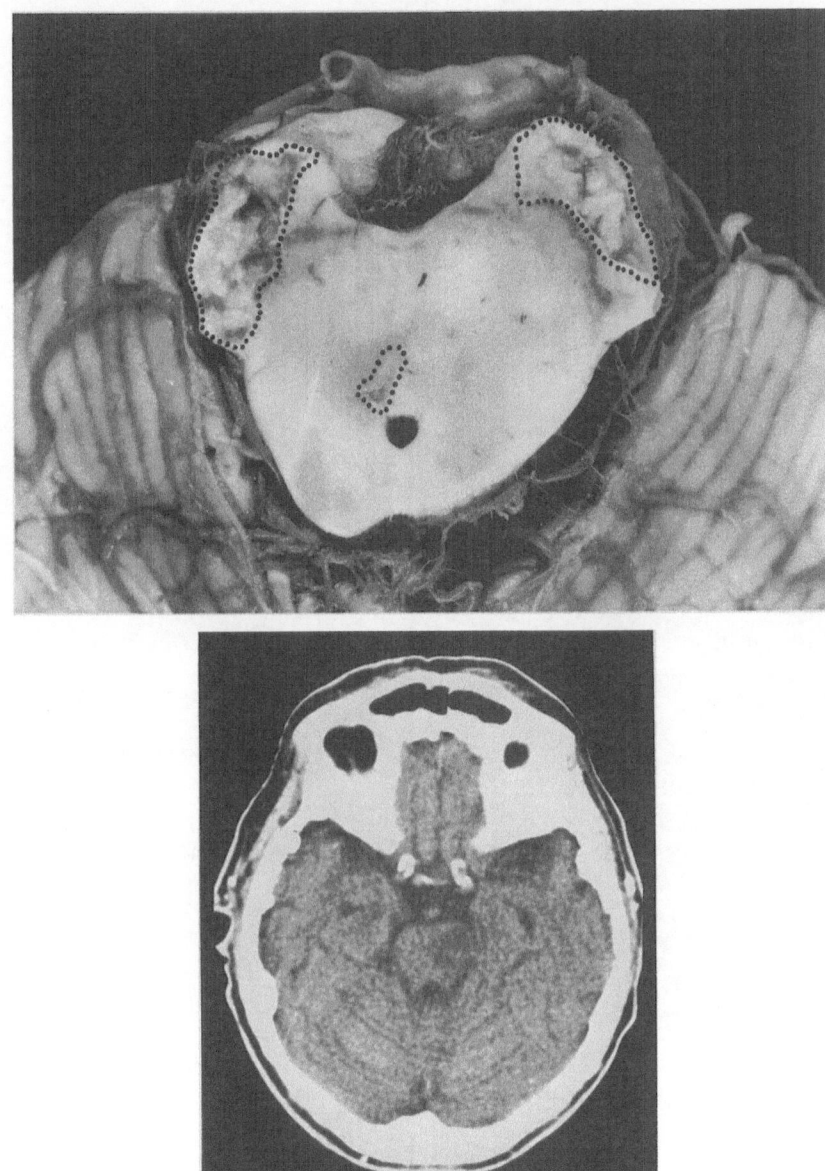

Fig. 52. a Bilateral totally necrotic infarcts of most of peduncular areas. Small lacunar cystic infarct in the periaqueductal gray. **b** Small infarct in peduncular and tectal area of mesencephalon

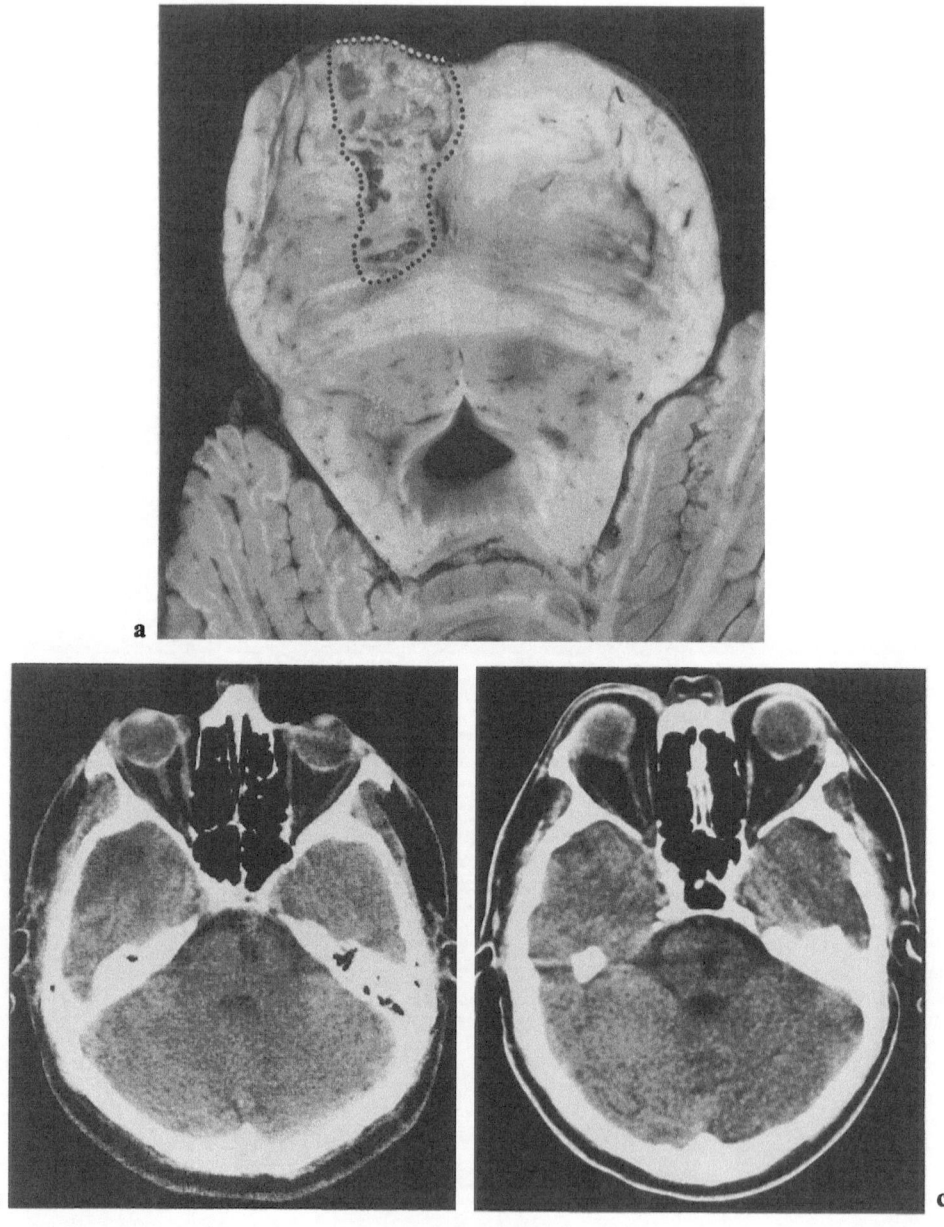

Fig. 53. a Cystic infarct in supply area of paramedian artery of pons. **b, c** Infarcts
of paramedian artery of pons

2.3.5.1 Infarct of the Paramedian Pontine Artery (Fig. 53a, b)

The paramedian infarct presents itself as a small zone reaching from the basis pontis to the tectum. Paramedian infarcts are frequently bilateral, are preferentially total, and rarely involve only the distal or proximal part of the irrigating area. There is occasionally in the pons a combination of infarcts of several arteries (Fig. 54a, b).

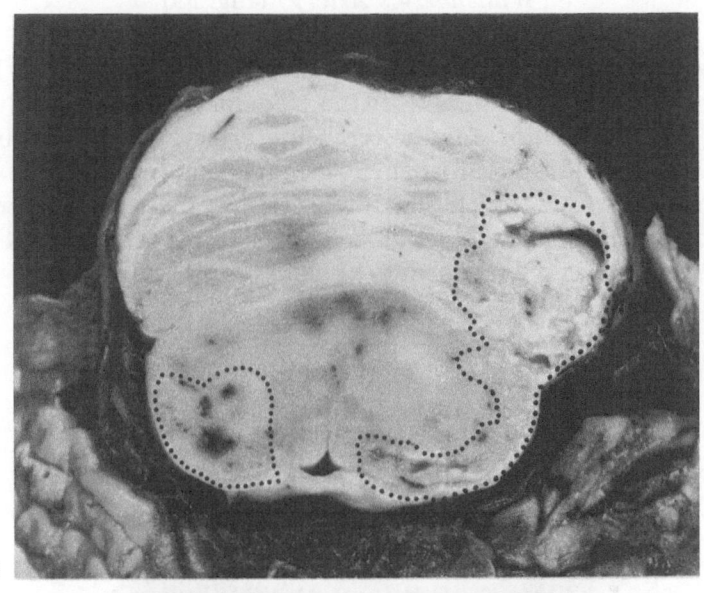

a

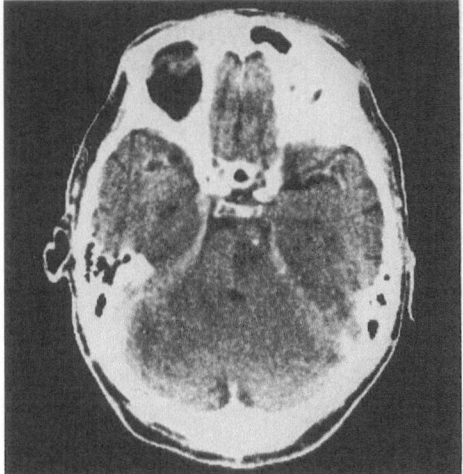

b

Fig. 54. a Large infarct showing beginning of cystic transformation in supply area of long circumflex artery of pons. Infarct extends into tectum. On the contralateral side a smaller infarct is seen only in the tectum. **b** Infarct of paramedian and short circumflex arteries of pons

2.3.5.2 *Infarct of the Long Circumflex Pontine Artery* (Fig. 54a)

The irrigating area of the artery is either totally or partially infarcted from its outer edge at the pons up to the tegmental area.

2.3.5.3 *Infarcts of the Posterior Inferior Cerebellar Artery (Wallenberg's Artery)* (Fig. 55)

These are infarcts which can be precisely localized clinically. The most typical is the dorsolateral infarct of the medulla oblongata resulting from occlusion of the posterior inferior cerebellar artery. The so-called Wallenberg syndrome can also occur when, as mentioned above, the artery consists of two small branches which separately irrigate the tonsillar area of the cerebellum and the medulla oblongata. This infarct is very difficult to recognize with certainty in CT scans.

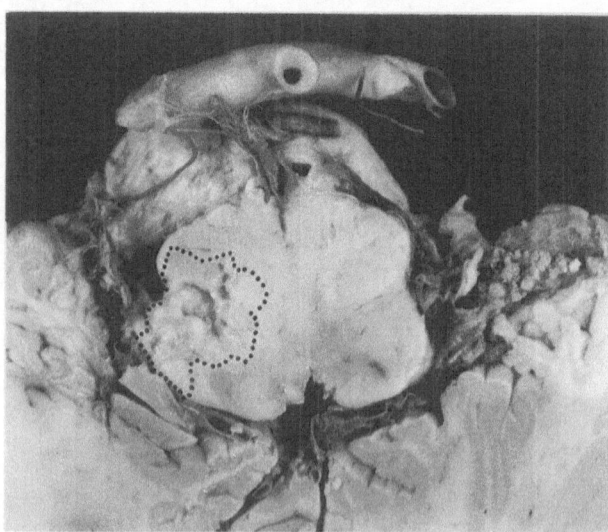

Fig. 55. Typical softened dorsolateral infarction of posterior inferior cerebellar artery (Wallenberg)

3 The Watershed (Border Zone) Infarcts

3.1 Annular Infarcts
(Figs. 56a, b; 57a, b; 60)

The curious lesion occurring between the irrigating areas of the middle cerebral artery on the one hand and the anterior and posterior cerebral arteries on the other has been known for a long time (since the studies of thromboangiitis obliterans of LINDENBERG and SPATZ 1940). The infarcted area there appears in the form of a granular atrophy (Figs. 59a, 60). The concept of the authors was that the thromboangiitic occlusion of the arteries would take place in this area preferentially and that the lesion would not be caused by a hemodynamic disturbance. However, this annular infarcted lesion can also be formed with open vessels, a fact we have observed not infrequently in pathological specimens. A crater-like lesion, deeply shrunken and grooved, is observed as a ring (Fig. 59a) around the territory of the middle cerebral artery (ZÜLCH 1981, Fig. 145).

We know from CT scans that this type of infarct can also be located in single divisions of the angular area only, more commonly in the frontal part. This has been emphasized by WODARZ (1975). However, morphologically, in the ideal case these annular infarcts may be formed on both sides: frontodorsal, parietal, and laterobasal (e.g., in the temporal area).

3.1.1 Annular Infarct of the Watersheds, Anterior Part
(Fig. 56a)

In partial infarction, one sees deep, shrunken grooves situated in the frontal portion of the watershed between the anterior and middle cerebral arteries. These lesions may be either unilateral or bilaterally symmetrical.

3.1.2 Annular Infarct of the Watersheds, Posterior Part
(Fig. 57a)

This watershed infarct presents itself at the border zone of the middle and posterior cerebral arteries in a laterobasal location. WODARZ et al. (1981) saw such border zone infarcts in association with carotid insufficiency in 40% of cases. Bilateral border zone infarcts were also described by FISHER and McQUILLEN (1981).

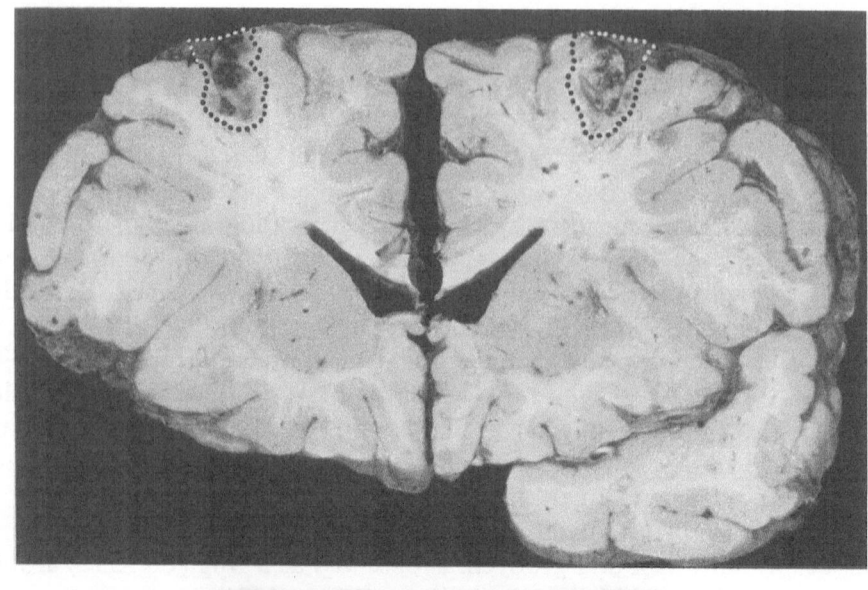

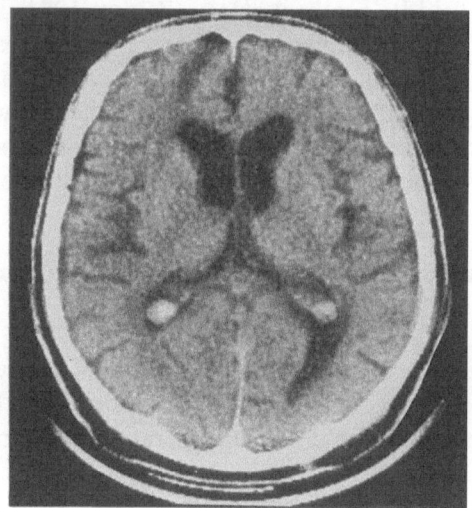

Fig. 56. a Circular border zone infarct in anterior third between the anterior cerebral and middle cerebral arteries, upper division. **b** Circular infarct of border zone (watershed), anterior division

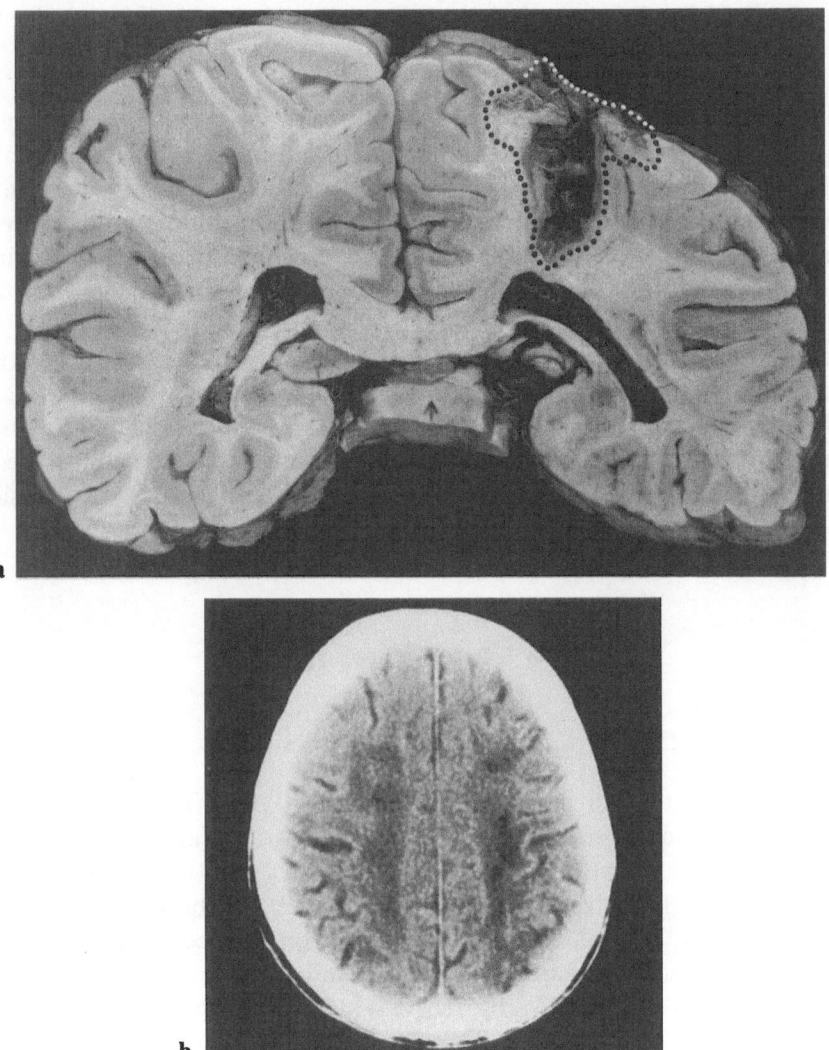

Fig. 57. a Circular border zone infarct on right side between middle cerebral artery (upper division) and anterior cerebral artery. It is deeply grooved and cystic. **b** Circular border zone infarcts, anterior and posterior division

3.1.3 Three-Territory Border Infarct (Dreiländereck-Infarkt)
(Fig. 58 a, b)

This infarct is by no means rare (see Zülch 1981, Fig. 149) and it cannot be explained by the concept of "terminal" infarction (e.g., of the posterior parietal or the angular artery). It is located in the area at the margin of the territories of the three principal cerebral arteries (middle, anterior, and posterior). At autopsy it is usually deep and shrunken or transformed into a cyst. It is not life-threatening. In CT scans it is usually seen when it is fresh.

The first observation of this anatomical pattern was made by J.E. Meyer (1953, 1958). He saw it with infantile vascular disorders as well as in atherosclerosis. This specific infarct is not uncommon with global ischemias, where it can be only explained on hemodynamic grounds. In the later stages it appears as a deep crater in the three-territory border, usually on one side, but it may (Fig. 58a) also be bilateral (Zülch 1981, Figs. 148 and 149).

4 The Multiinfarct Brain
(Fig. 59 a–c)

This spotty pattern of small infarcts has been described in anatomical specimens. It is usually accompanied by a psychiatric syndrome with disturbance of cognitive function. Therefore, the term "multiinfarct dementia" (Hachinski et al. 1974; Zeumer and Hacke 1982) has been used. One can often observe in CT scans of elderly persons the presence of multiple small infarcts which are either isolated or connected by a broad band of small scars, so-called granular atrophy (see Figs. 5d, 59a, p. 60). This picture will be encountered frequently in CT scans from psychiatric hospitals where there are many demented patients.

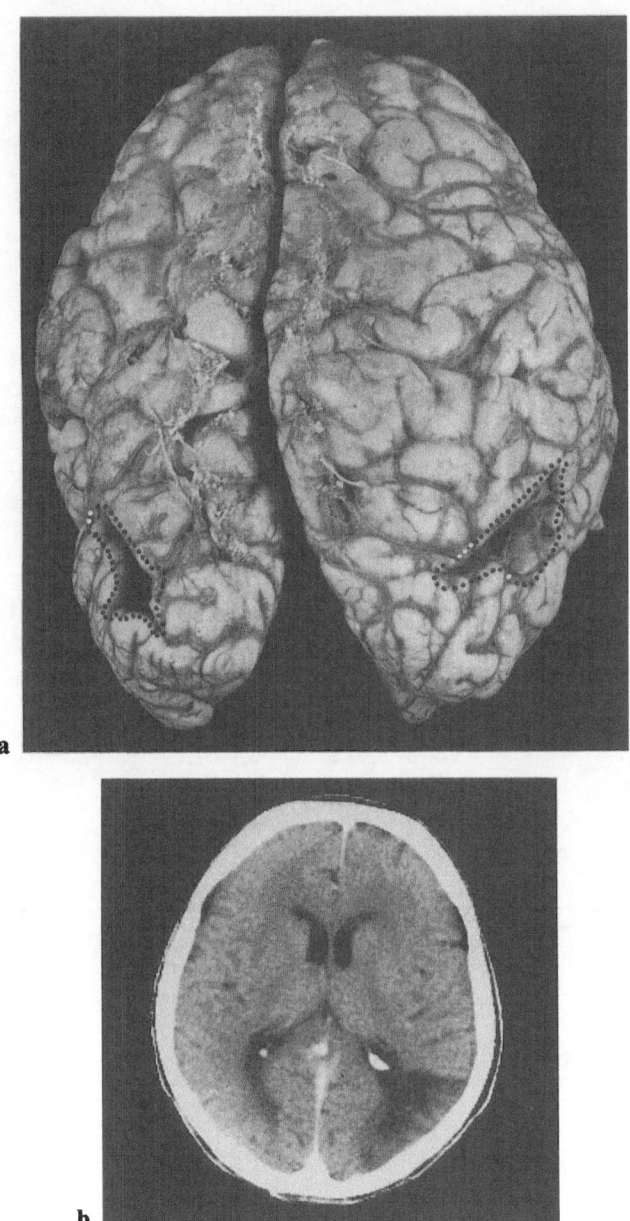

Fig. 58. a Bilateral, **b** unilateral "three-territory infarct"

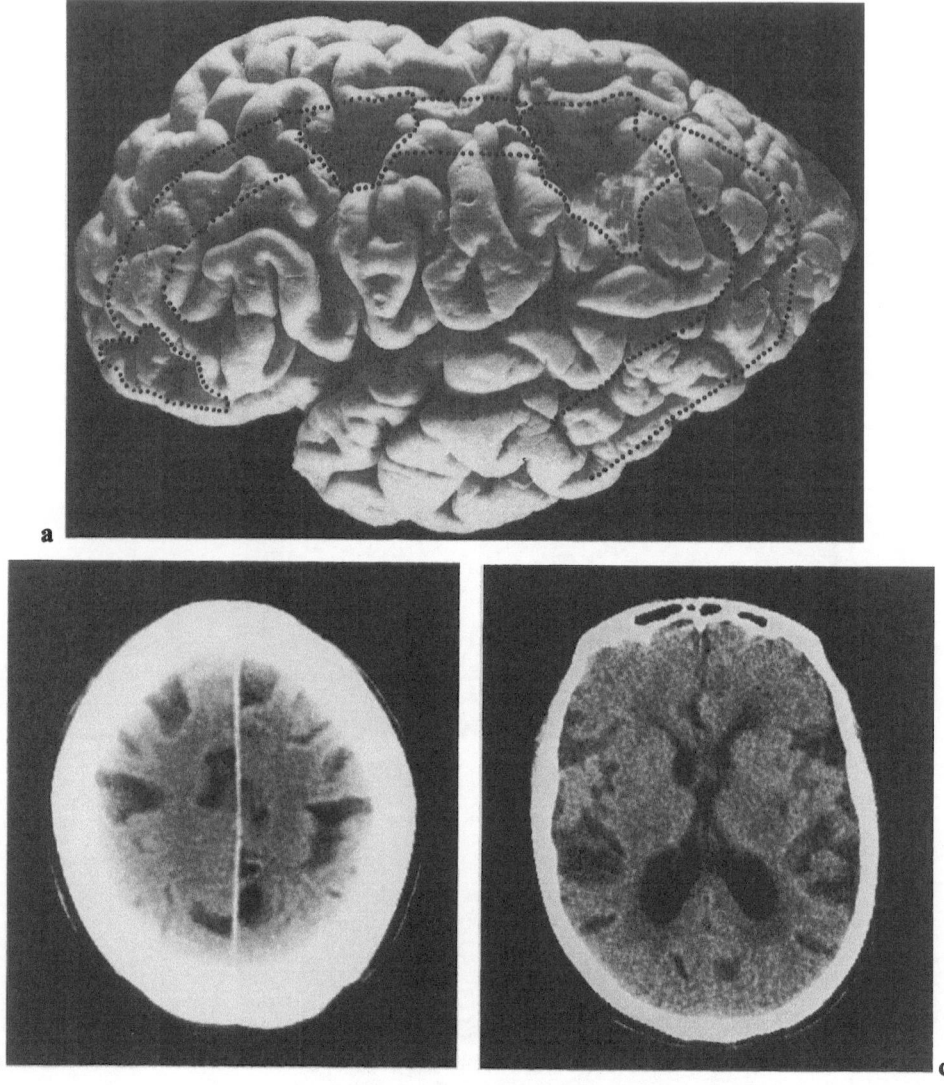

Fig. 59. a Multiple crater-like unsystematic infarction scars: so-called multiinfarct brain. Incomplete circular infarction zone of granular atrophy can be seen. **b, c** Multiinfarct brains in CT scan

5 Atrophic Processes: Ischemic Atrophies
(Fig. 43a, b)

Atrophy of the aged has a certain regional predilection. It usually involves the frontal and frontotemporal convolutions first and then later the centro-parietal area (see Fig. 43a). This process is manifested in the CT scan by widening of the sulci. It must be emphasized that some parts of the brain are spared by this atrophic process, namely the fronto-orbital cortex, the temporobasal parts, and the entire occipital lobe. Therefore, if one finds widening of the sulci there or in the occipital area, the atrophic process cannot be part of an atrophy of the aged (see Fig. 43a, b).

On the other hand, Alzheimer's atrophy, now so often discussed and investigated, extends over the entire brain, with only the temporomedial part of the hippocampus and uncus area rarely being less involved for some time. Alzheimer's disease can readily be recognized by this distribution pattern.

Pick's atrophy has a regional predilection for the frontal lobe, including the fronto-orbital portion, which is usually spared in the atrophy of the aged. It can also be localized to the temporal lobe including involvement of the basal parts, which are also spared in atrophy of the aged. A parietal location of Pick's atrophy is seen only rarely.

We will not go into detail here but merely mention other atrophic disorders (MEESE and GRUMME 1980), such as Huntington's disease and Binswanger's disease (DE REUCK et al. 1980; ZEUMER et al. 1980), thromboangiitis obliterans (ZÜLCH 1969; Fig. 60).

In the atrophic process of aging, the cortex is sometimes more involved, while in other cases it may be the white matter, or both, so that one finds

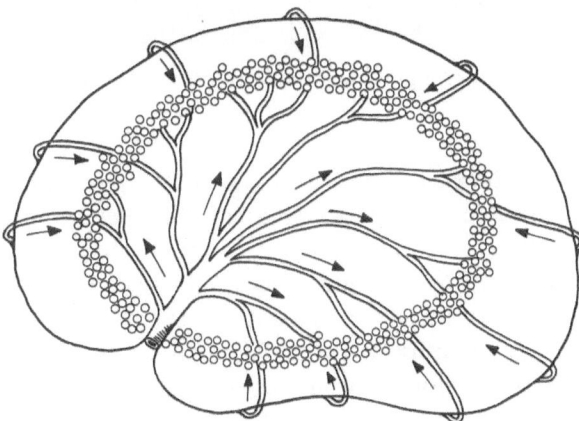

Fig. 60. Schematic drawing of circular zone of granular atrophy in thromboangiitis obliterans due to relative ischemia in the most distant fields

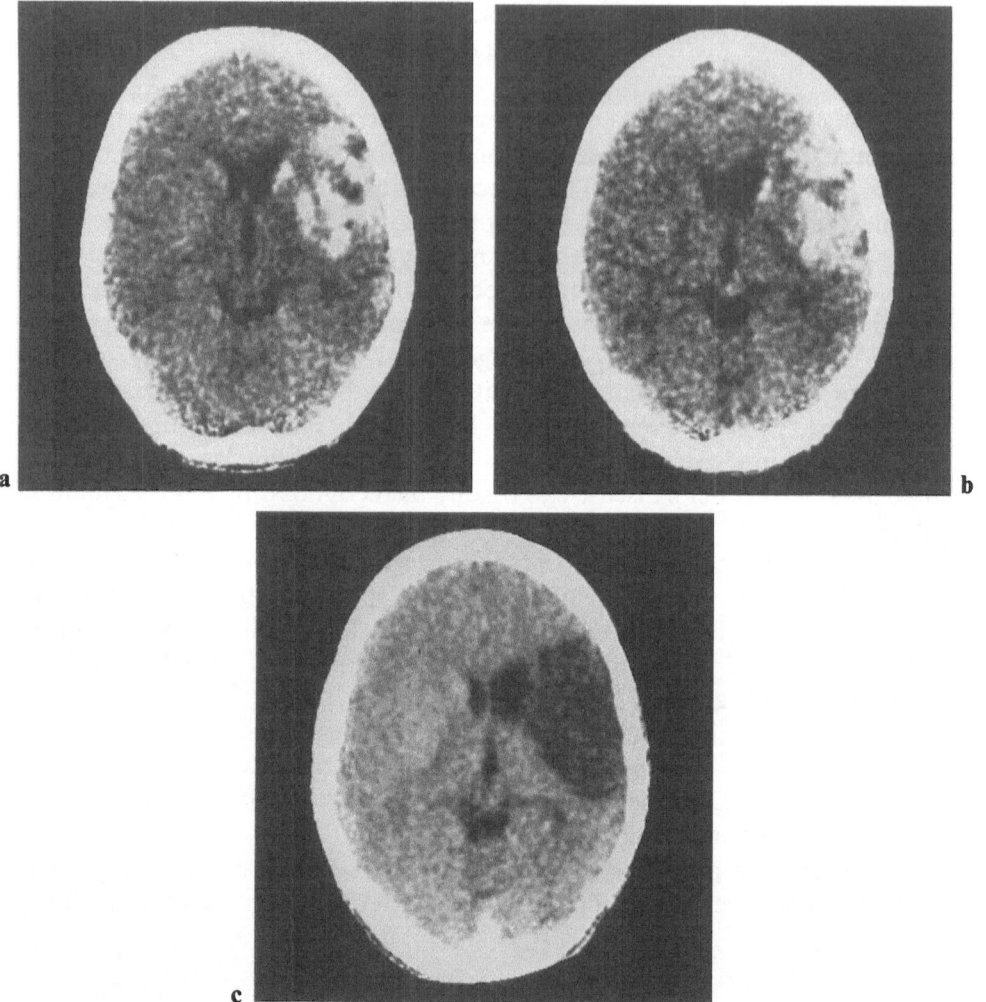

Fig. 61. a, b Typical hemorrhagic infarct. **c** Huge cyst 9 months later, same infarct

either a more pronounced dilatation of the sulci or an enlargement of the ventricles. A reasonable explanation for this difference is not known. At the same time, no explanation has been found for why we have regional preferences in the atrophy of aging, particularly for the frontotemporal or the centroparietal areas. In any event, as far as we can deduce up to the present time, the atrophy of the aged, in the majority of cases, is not of vascular origin, but a biological process of its own. This does not contradict the finding when one uses regional blood flow measurements that there are typical atrophies based on regional vascular deficiencies (see INGVAR 1977).

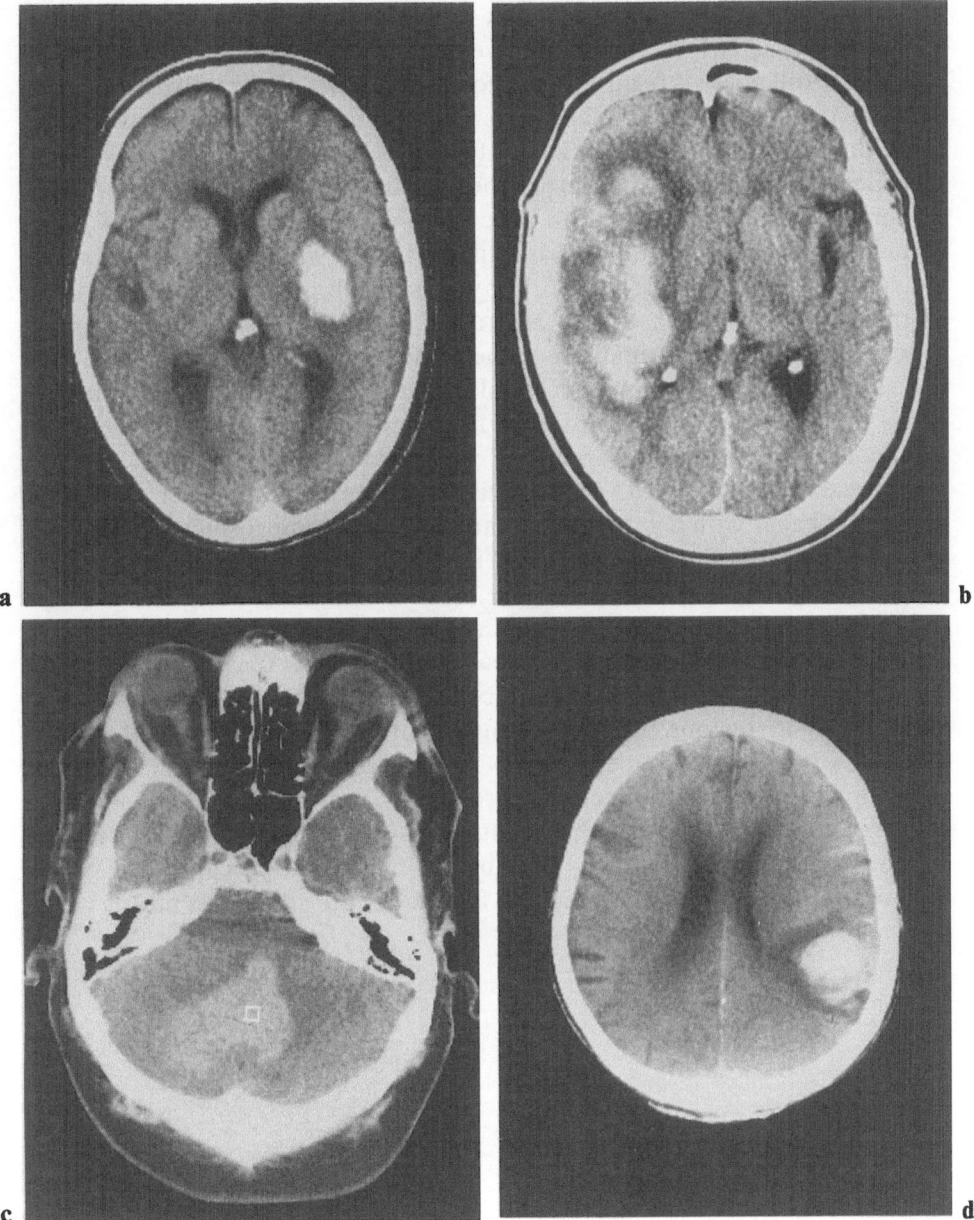

Fig. 62. a Relatively small typical mass hemorrhage which has not ruptured into ventricle. **b** Large mass hemorrhage extending into frontal and temporal lobe. **c** Typical large cerebellar mass hemorrhage. **d** Small atypical mass hemorrhage, subcortically situated in temporo-occipital area

For CT scans it has been said that the width of the sulci must be below 0.5 cm. All cases where this figure is exceeded are pathological. Moreover, discussion still goes on regarding the correspondence of the ventricular width to a particular age-group. One must recognize that after approximately the 25th year, the weight of the brain steadily decreases, as shown in excellent statistical measurements collected close to the beginning of the nineteenth century (ZÜLCH 1983). This can occur naturally only as a result of a loss of brain substance, beginning particularly in the white matter. Years ago, we designed a series of schematic drawings which are useful only as a rule of thumb (ZÜLCH 1950, Fig. 4; KAUTZKY et al. 1982, Fig. 180), according to which the greatest normal size of the ventricles can be determined. Similar measurements of the pneumoencephalogram were attempted over many decades (for instance by SCHIERSMANN 1952 and HUBER 1957) and they have been confirmed in recent years by CT in a particular age group.

These data are of great significance because the evaluation of the CT scan must begin with a general comparison of the cerebrospinal fluid spaces with the figures defined as "normal" for the corresponding age.

This is equally important for the evaluation of the CT scan in brain infarcts. In a great number of cases, an additional atrophic process of the aged or, in contrast, a general global ischemic (vascular) atrophy of the brain may exist. Ischemic origin can be accepted in any case where atrophy is observed in regions which are usually preserved (see above) from the atrophic process in the aged (BARRON et al. 1976).

Atrophies observed in alcoholics are also of importance. They have been observed in 44% of their alcoholic patients by STROBL et al. (1980). According to CARLEN et al. (1978) they may be reversible in some cases. The pathogenesis and pattern of the atrophy in alcoholics are still by no means clear.

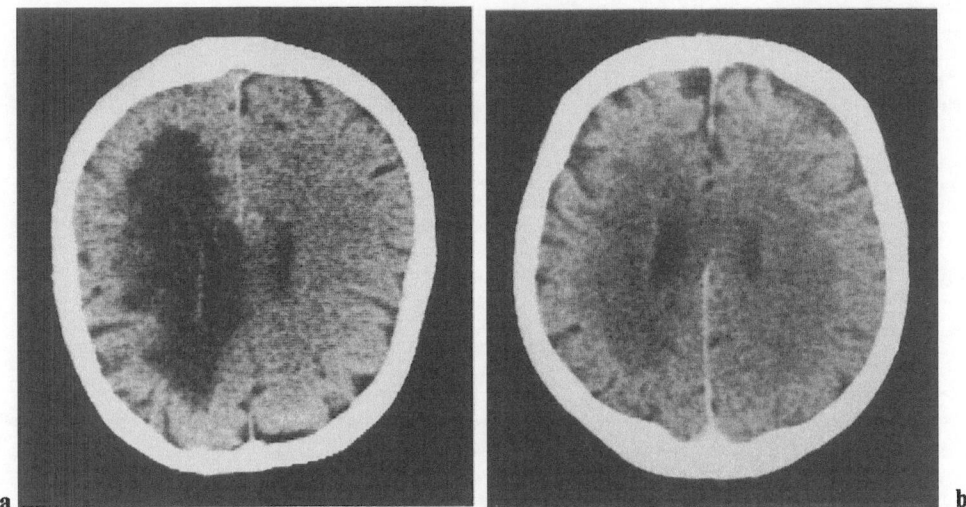

a   b

Fig. 63. a Gross edema formation in right hemisphere after an acute hypertensive crisis. **b** Regression of edema 2 weeks later with only minor lesions of the myelin

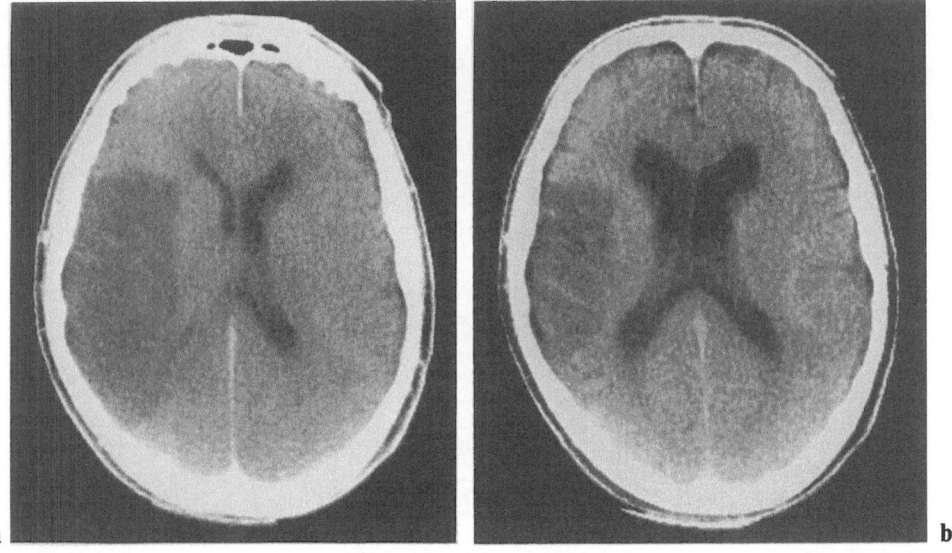

a   b

Fig. 64. a Fresh (2nd day) infarction in medial supply area of middle cerebral artery. **b** Three months later CT scan shows necrosis in infarcted area reaching down into basal parts

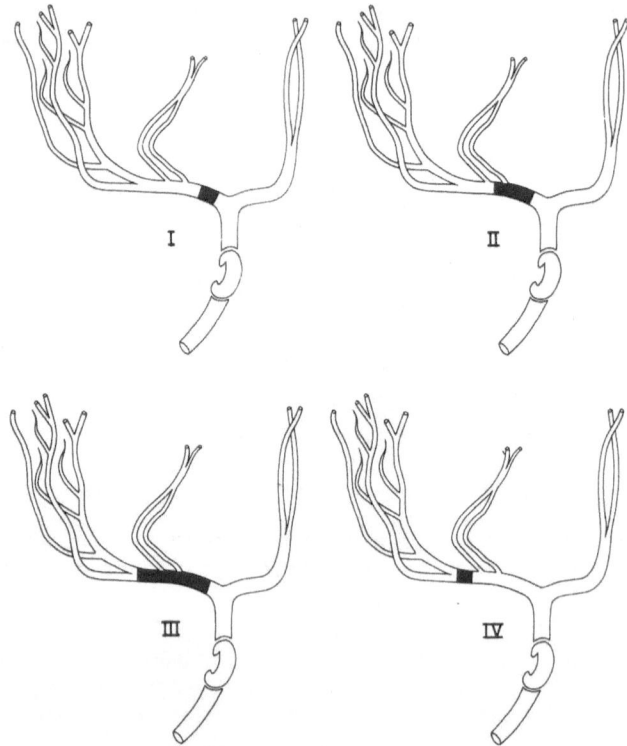

Fig. 65. Four predilection sites for atherosclerotic occlusions of middle cerebral artery: *I*, proximal location; *II*, proximal occlusion extending to origin of medial striate arteries; *III*, proximal occlusion of all striate arteries; and *IV*, distal occlusion

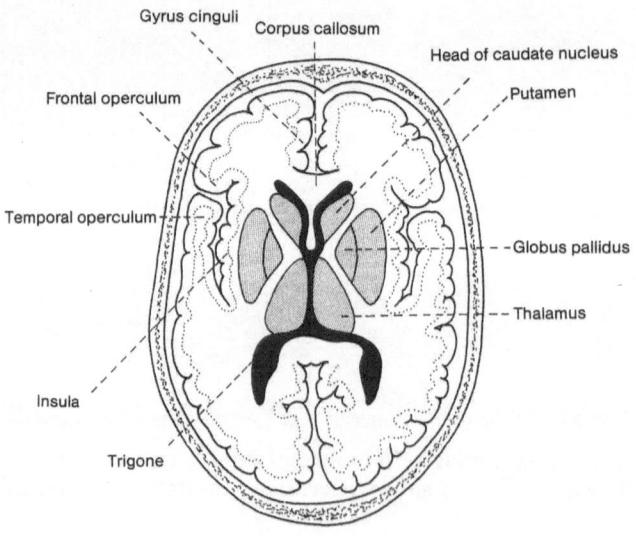

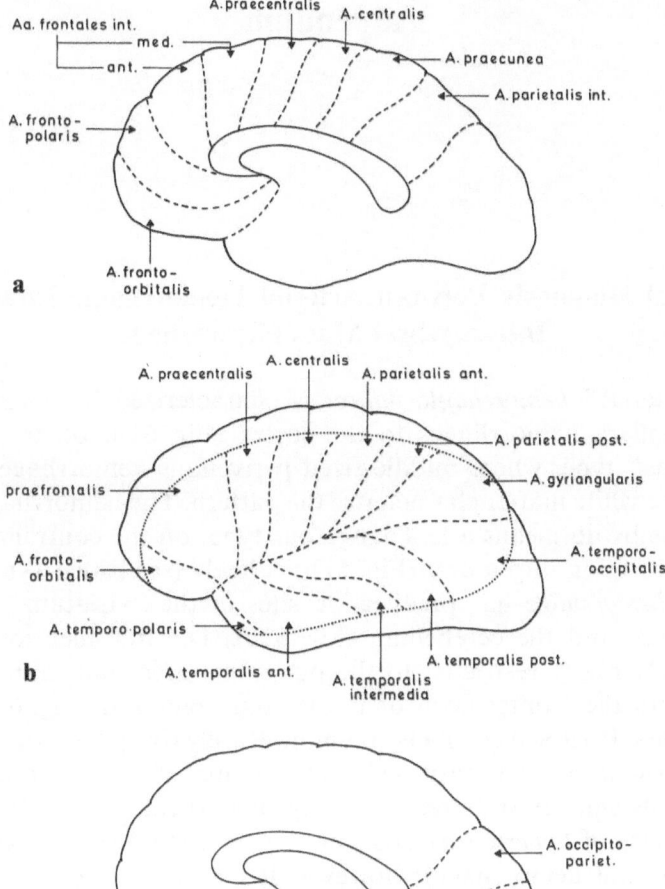

Fig. 67. The terminal branches and supply areas of the three main cerebral source arteries [anterior (**a**), middle (**b**), and posterior (**c**) cerebral arteries]. The terminology of the terminal branches of the three great cerebral arteries is chaotically inconsistent. I have attempted to select the most informative terms from the books and atlases of FOIX and LEY (1927), KRAYENBÜHL and YASARGIL (1965), SALAMON and HUANG (1976), and NADJMI and RATZKA (1981)

Fig. 66. Topographical drawing of the most important regions mentioned in the text

Addendum

Differential Diagnosis Between Arterial Hemorrhagic Infarction and Intracerebral Mass Hemorrhage

The "arterial" *hemorrhagic infarct* is characterized by a restriction of the pericapillary hemorrhages to the cortex (Fig. 61 a, b), in contrast to the "venous" type, where middle sized perivenous hemorrhages predominantly in the white matter characterize the pattern. The hemorrhagic ("red") infarction is by no means a less dangerous type; on the contrary, organization and transition into a cyst (Fig. 61 b) is likely (see Zülch 1981, p. 84 ff.). The *mass hemorrhage* has predilection sites in the "striatum" (Fig. 62 a), the thalamus, and the cerebellum (Fig. 62 c). The first-mentioned hemorrhage is only rarely restricted to the putaminal area, but more frequently ruptures into the frontal horn or the frontal, temporal (Fig. 62 b), and/or parietal lobes. Perifocal edema is common. Rarely (frequency of about 10%) the hemorrhage has an "atypical" site in one of the neighboring lobes and is usually smaller and predominantly subcortical (Fig. 62 d).

The sequelae of *hypertensive crisis* may be manyfold (for instance triggering of a striatal hemorrhage); however, it may also lead to an extensive subcortical edema, which may be resolved later (Fig. 63 a) without much destruction of white matter.

Prognosis. As demonstrated in Fig. 63 a, b it is difficult to prognosticate the sequelae of an edematous "infarction"; Fig. 64 a, b is an example of such a wrong prognosis (see p. 19).

Sufficient information on the different types of pathogenesis of middle cerebral artery occlusion is provided in Fig. 65. Despite "occlusion" of the source artery, the ensuing infarcts may be different (Zülch 1981, p. 132 ff.) in size and location.

Figures 66 and 67 were added to facilitate orientation without extensive searching in various atlases.

References

Adams AE, Rosenberger K, Winter H, Zöllner C (1977) A case of cortical deafness. Arch Psychiatr Nervenkr 224:213–220

Alcalá H, Gado M, Torack RM (1978) The effect of size, histologic elements, and water content on the visualization of cerebral infarcts. Arch Neurol 35:1–7

Aulich A, Fenske A (1977) Das Computer-Tomogramm des Schlaganfalles. Aktuel Neurol 4:129–140

Aulich A, Wende S, Fenske A, Lange S, Steinhoff H (1976) Diagnosis and follow-up studies in cerebral infarcts. In: Lanksch W, Kazner E (eds) Cranial computerized tomography. Springer, Berlin Heidelberg New York, pp 273–283

Barron SA, Jacobs L, Kinkel WR (1976) Changes in size of normal lateral ventricles during aging determined by computerized tomography. Neurology (Minneap) 26:1011–1013

Becker H, Desch H, Hacker H, Pencz A (1979) CT fogging effect with ischemic cerebral infarcts. Neuroradiology 18:185–192

Botton J (1955) Artériosclérose cérébrale. Etude anatomo-clinique et statistique. Thèse de Genève. Doin, Paris

Büchner F (1939) Die Coronarinsuffizienz. Steinkopff, Dresden

Büchner F (1964) Struktur, Stoffwechsel und Funktion in der modernen Pathologie, Vorträge und Vorlesungen in Japan. Urban and Schwarzenberg, München

Carlen PL, Wortzman G, Holgate RC, Wilkinson DA, Rankin JG (1978) Reversible cerebral atrophy in recently abstinent chronic alcoholics measured by computed tomography scans. Science 200:1076–1078

Cohnheim J (1882) Vorlesungen über allgemeine Pathologie, vol I, 2nd edn. Hirschwald, Berlin

Cooper IS (1956) The neurosurgical alleviation of Parkinsonism. Thomas, Springfield

Corday E, Rothenberg SF (1957) The clinical aspects of cerebral vascular insufficiency. Ann Intern Med 47:626–639

Cronqvist S, Brismar J, Kjellin K, Sönderström CE (1975) Computer assisted axial tomography in cerebrovascular lesions. Acta Radiol (Diagn) (Stockh) 16:135–145

De Reuck J, Crevitis L, Decoster S, Sieben B, Van der Eecken H (1980) Pathogenesis of Binswager's chronic progressive subcortical encephalopathy. Neurology (NY) 30:920–928

Earnest MP, Monroe PA, Yarnell PR (1977) Cortical deafness: demonstration of the pathologic anatomy by CT scan. Neurology (Minneap) 27:1172–1175

Einsiedel-Lechtape H, Kleihues P (1977) Pathology of cerebral vascular insufficiency. In: Hewton TH, Potts DG (eds) Radiology of the skull and brain, vol III. Mosby, St Louis, pp 3173–3196

Fischer-Brügge E (1949) Der persistierende Hirnprolaps nach Schußverletzungen. Zentralbl Neurochir 9:18–45

Fisher CM (1951) Occlusion of the internal carotid artery. Arch Neurol Psychiatry 65:346

Fisher CM (1965) Lacunes: small deep cerebral infarcts. Neurology (Minneap) 15:774–784

Fisher CM (1967) A lacunar stroke. The dysarthria-clumsy hand syndrome. Neurology (Minneap) 17:614–617

Fisher CM (1969) The arterial lesions underlying lacunes. Acta Neuropathol (Berl) 12:1–15

Fisher CM (1971) Pathologic observations in hypertensive cerebral hemorrhage. J Neuropathol Exp Neurol 30:536–550

Fisher M, McQuillen JB (1981) Bilateral cortical borderzone infarction. A pseudo-brainstem stroke. Arch Neurol 38:62–63

Foix C, Ley J (1927) Contribution à l'étude du ramollissement cérébral envisagé au point de vue de sa fréquence, de son siège et de l'état anatomique des artères du territoire nécrosé. J Neurol (Brux) 27:658–684

Hachinski VC, Lassen NA, Marshall J (1974) Multi-infarct dementia. A cause of mental deterioration in the elderly. Lancet II:207–209

Hammer B (1982) Soll beim CT des Hirninfarktes Kontrastmittel gegeben werden? 3rd neuroradiological contrast medium symposium, Boppard

Hayman LA, Evans RA, Hinck VC (1979) Rapid high dose (RHD) contrast cranial computed tomography: a concise review of normal anatomy. J Comput Assist Tomogr 3:147–154

Heubner O (1872) Zur Topographie der Ernährungsgebiete der einzelnen Hirnarterien. Zentralbl Med Wiss 10:817–821

Heubner O (1874) Die luetische Erkrankung der Hirnarterien. Vogel, Leipzig

Hirsch H, Schneider M (1968) Durchblutung und Sauerstoffaufnahme des Gehirns. In: Olivecrona H, Tönnis W (eds) Chemischer Aufbau, Physiologie, Pathophysiologie. Springer, Berlin Heidelberg New York, pp 434–552 (Handbuch der Neurochirurgie, vol I/2)

Huber G (1957) Pneumencephalographische und psychopathologische Bilder bei endogenen Psychosen. Springer, Berlin Göttingen Heidelberg

Huber G, Emde H, Piepgras U (1978) Der raumfordernde anaemische Hirninfarkt im cerebralen Computertomogramm. Nervenarzt 49:417–421

Ingvar DH (1977) Distribution of cerebral blood flow at rest and during mental activation in normals and in patients with brain disorders. In: Zülch KJ, Kaufmann W, Hossmann K-A, Hossmann V (eds) Brain and heart infarct. Springer, Berlin Heidelberg New York, pp 167–174

Kautzky R, Zülch KJ, Wende S, Tänzer A (1976) Neuroradiologie auf neuropathologischer Grundlage. Springer, Berlin Heidelberg New York

Kautzky R, Zülch KJ, Wende S, Tänzer A (1982) Neuroradiology. A neuropathological approach. Springer, Berlin Heidelberg New York

Kawase T, Mizukami M, Araki G (1981) Mechanisms of contrast enhancement in cerebral infarction: computerized tomography, regional cerebral blood flow, fluorescein angiography, and pathological study. Adv Neurol 30:149–158

Kazner E, Wende S, Grumme T, Lanksch W, Stochdorph O (1981) Computertomographie intrakranieller Tumoren aus klinischer Sicht. Springer, Berlin Heidelberg New York

Kleihues P (1966) Isolierte Infarkte in der Sehstrahlung. Albrecht Von Graefes Arch Klin Exp Ophthalmol 169:181–193

Kleihues P, Hizawa K (1966) Die Infarkte der A. cerebri posterior: Pathogenese und topographische Beziehungen zur Sehrinde. Arch Psychiatr Nervenkr 208:263–284

Kohlmeyer K, Graser C (1978a) Comparative study of computed tomography (CCT) and carotid angiography (CAG) in stroke patients. Neuroradiology 16:162–163

Kohlmeyer K, Graser C (1978b) Comparative studies of computed tomography and measurements of regional blood flow in stroke patients. Neuroradiology 16:233–237

Krayenbühl H, Yasargil MG (1965) Die zerebrale Angiographie, 2nd edn. Thieme, Stuttgart

Kribs M, Kleihues P (1971) The recurrent artery of Heubner. A morphological study of the blood supply of the rostral basal ganglia in normal and pathological conditions. In: Zülch KJ (ed) Cerebral circulation and stroke. Springer, Berlin Heidelberg New York, pp 40–56

Kubik CS, Adams RD (1946) Occlusion of the basilar artery. A clinical and pathological study. Brain 69:73–121

Lang J (1981) Klinische Anatomie des Kopfes. Neurokranium, Orbita, kraniozervikaler Übergang. Springer, Berlin Heidelberg New York

Lee KF, Chambers RA, Diamond C, Park CH, Thompson NL Jr, Schnapf D, Pripstein S (1978) Evaluation of cerebral infarction by computed tomography with special emphasis on microinfarction. Neuroradiology 16:156–158

Levine DN, Mohr JP (1979) Language after bilateral cerebral infarctions: role of the minor hemisphere in speech. Neurology (Minneap) 29:927–938

Lindenberg R, Spatz H (1940) Über die Thromboendarteriitis obliterans der Hirngefäße (cerebrale Form der v. Winiwarter-Buergerschen Krankheit). Virchows Arch [Pathol Anat] 305:531–557

Manelfe C, Clonet M, Gigaud M, Bonafe A, Guiraud B, Rascol A (1981) Internal capsule: normal anatomy and ischemic changes demonstrated by computed tomography. AJNR 2:149–155

Masdeu JC, Azar-Kia B, Rubino FA (1977) Evaluation of recent cerebral infarction by computerized tomography. Arch Neurol 34:417–421

Meese W, Grumme T (1980) Die Beurteilung hirnatrophischer Prozesse mit Hilfe der Computertomographie. Fortschr Neurol 48:494–509

Meyer JE (1953) Über die Lokalisation frühkindlicher Hirnschäden in arteriellen Grenzgebieten. Arch Psychiatr Nervenkr 190:328–341

Meyer JE (1958) Zur Lokalisation arteriosklerotischer Erweichungsherde in arteriellen Grenzgebieten des Gehirns. Arch Psychiatr Nervenkr 196:421–432

Moore MT, Stern K (1938) Vascular lesion in brain-stem and occipital lobe occurring in association with brain tumors. Brain 61:70–98

Müller HR (1979) The place of computerized tomography and carotid Doppler sonography in CV episodes. Adv Neurol 25:181–197

Nadjmi M, Ratzka M (1981) Normale Anatomie der cerebralen Arterien. In: Diethelm L, Wende S (eds) Roentgendiagnosis of the central nervous system. Springer, Berlin Heidelberg New York, pp 327–416 (Handbuch der medizinischen Radiologie, vol XIV, part 1A)

Norton GA, Kishore PRS, Lin J (1978) CT contrast enhancement in cerebral infarction. Am J Roentgenol 131:881–885

Okuno T, Takao T, Ito M, Konishi Y, Mikawa H, Nakano Y (1980) Infarction of the internal capsule in children. J Comput Assist Tomogr 4:770–774

Opitz E, Schneider M (1950) Über die Sauerstoffversorgung des Gehirns und den Mechanismus von Mangelwirkungen. Ergeb Physiol 46:126–260

Ostertag CB, Mundinger F (1978) Diagnostic errors in the interpretation of cerebral infarction. Adv Neurosurg 6:86–89

Ostertag CB, Unsöld R (1981) Korrelation computertomographisch dargestellter Infarkte der Sehrinde mit homonymen Gesichtsfeldausfällen. Arch Psychiatr Nervenkr 230:265–274

Pernkopf E (1957) Topographische Anatomie des Menschen, vol IV. Topographische und stratigraphische Anatomie des Kopfes, erste Hälfte. Urban and Schwarzenberg, München

Pernkopf E (1960) Topographische Anatomie des Menschen, vol IV. Topographische und stratigraphische Anatomie des Kopfes, zweite Hälfte. Urban and Schwarzenberg, München

Pfeifer RA (1930) Grundlegende Untersuchungen über die Angioarchitektonik des menschlichen Gehirns. Springer, Berlin

Pfeifer RA (1931) Anastomosen der Hirngefäße, dargestellt am asphyktisch-hyperämischen Kindergehirn. J Psychol Neurol (Leipz) 42:1–173

Pullicino P, Kendall BE (1980) Contrast enhancement in ischaemic lesions. Neuroradiology 19:235–239

Pullicino P, Nelson RF, Kendall BE, Marshall J (1980) Small deep infarcts diagnosed on computed tomography. Neurology (NY) 30:1090–1096

Radü EW, Moseley IF (1978) Carotid artery occlusion and computed tomography. Neuroradiology 17:7–12

Rail DL, Perkin GD (1980) Computerized tomographic appearance of hypertensive encephalopathy. Arch Neurol 37:310–311

Rein H (1931) Die Physiologie der Coronardurchblutung. Verh Dtsch Ges Inn Med 43:247–262

Rein H (1936) Einführung in die Physiologie des Menschen. Springer, Berlin

Riessner D, Zülch KJ (1939) Über die Formveränderungen des Hirns (Massenverschiebungen, Zisternenverquellungen) bei raumbeengenden Prozessen. Dtsch Z Chir 253:1–61

Salamon G (1971) Atlas de la vascularisation artérielle du cerveau chez l'homme. Sandoz, Paris

Salamon G, Huang YP (1976) Radiologic anatomy of the brain. Springer, Berlin Heidelberg New York

Schiersmann O (1952) Einführung in die Encephalographie. Thieme, Stuttgart

Schmidt HW (1955) Über Arterienkreise in der Pia mater des Menschen. Dtsch Z Nervenheilk 172:526–530

Schneider M (1951) Kreislauf und Gehirn. Steinkopf, Dresden

Schneider M (1952) Chemie und Stoffwechsel der Nervengewebe. Mosbacher Colloquium. Springer, Berlin Göttingen Heidelberg

Skriver EB, Olsen TS (1982) Contrast enhancement of cerebral infarcts. Incidence and clinical value in different states of cerebral infarction. Neuroradiology 23:259–265

Steinhoff H, Ambrose J (1981) Computertomographie des Gehirns. In: Diethelm L, Heuck F, Olsson O, Strnad F, Vieten H, Zuppinger A (eds) Roentgendiagnosis of the central nervous system. Springer, Berlin Heidelberg New York, pp 269–415 (Handbuch der medizinischen Radiologie, vol XIV, part 1B)

Steinhoff H, Kazner E, Lanksch W, Grumme T, Meese W, Lange S, Aulich A, Wende S (1976) The limitations of computerized axial tomography in the detection and differential diagnosis of intracranial tumors. A study based on 1304 neoplasms. In: Boris J (ed) The diagnostic limitations of computerized axial tomography. Springer, Berlin Heidelberg New York, pp 40–49

Strobl G, Reisner T, Zeiler K (1980) Die craniale Computer-Tomographie in der Psychiatrie. Nervenarzt 51:36–40

Traupe H, Heiss WD, Hoeffken W, Zülch KJ (1979) Hyperfusion and enhancement in dynamic computed tomography of ischemic stroke patients. J Comput Assist Tomogr 3:627–632

Valk J (1980) Computed tomography and cerebral infarction. Lemniscaat, Rotterdam

Van den Bergh R (1969) The periventricular intracerebral blood supply. In: Meyer JS, Lechner H, Eichhorn O (eds) Research on the cerebral circulation. Thomas, Springfield, pp 52–65

Van der Eecken HM, Adams RD (1953) The anatomy and functional significance of the meningeal arterial anastomoses of the human brain. J Neuropathol Exp Neurol 12:132–157

Wing SD, Norman D, Pollock JA, Newton TH (1976) Contrast enhancement of cerebral infarcts in computed tomography. Radiology 121:89–92

Wodarz R (1975) Mediaastverschlüsse – 41 Fälle mit angiographischer, szintigraphischer und elektroenzephalographischer Korrelation zum klinischen Befund. Dissertation, University of Cologne

Wodarz R (1980) Watershed infarctions and computed tomography. A topographical study in cases with stenosis or occlusion of the carotid artery. Neuroradiology 19:245–248

Wodarz R, Ratzka M, Grosse D (1981) Der Grenzzoneninfarkt als besondere Infarktkonstellation bei Karotisinsuffizienz. Fortschr Röntgenstr 134:128–131

Yock DH, Marshall WH (1975) Recent ischemic brain infarcts at computed tomography: appearances pre- and postcontrast infusion. Radiology 117:599–608

Zeumer H, Hacke W (1982) Zur Frage der Multiinfarktdemenz unter besonderer Berücksichtigung computertomographischer Befunde. Fortschr Neurol Psychiatr 50:366–367

Zeumer H, Schonsky B, Sturm KW (1980) Predominant white matter involvement in subcortical arteriosclerotic encephalopathy (Binswanger's disease). J Comput Assist Tomogr 4:14–19

Zeumer H, Ringelstein EB, Klose KC (1981) Lakunäre Infarkte im Computertomogramm. Angiographische und differentialdiagnostische Gesichtspunkte. Fortschr Röntgenstr 134:488–494

Zülch KJ (1950) Röntgendiagnostik beim cerebralen Anfall. Verh Dtsch Ges Inn Med 56:24–48

Zülch KJ (1953) Neue Befunde und Deutungen aus der Gefäßpathologie des Hirns und Rückenmarks. Zentralbl Allg Pathol 90:402

Zülch KJ (1954) Mangeldurchblutung an der Grenzzone zweier Gefäßgebiete als Ursache bisher ungeklärter Rückenmarksschädigungen. Dtsch Z Nervenheilk 172:81–101

Zülch KJ (1959) Störungen des intrakraniellen Druckes. In: Olivecrona H, Tönnis W (eds) Angewandte Anatomie, Physiologie, Pathophysiologie. Springer, Berlin Göttingen Heidelberg, pp 208–303 (Handbuch der Neurochirurgie, vol I/1)

Zülch KJ (1961) Die Pathogenese von Massenblutung und Erweichung unter besonderer Berücksichtigung klinischer Gesichtspunkte. Acta Neurochir (Wien) Suppl VII:51–117

Zülch KJ (1968) The morphologic basis of the abnormal echo-encephalogram. In: Kazner E, Schiefer W, Zülch KJ (eds) Proceedings in echoencephalography. Springer, Berlin Heidelberg New York, pp 12–24

Zülch KJ (1969) The cerebral form of von Winiwarter-Buerger's disease: Does it exist? Angiology 20:61–69

Zülch KJ (1979) Predilection of cerebral atherosclerotic stenosis: a morphological and radiologic demonstration. In: Zülch KJ, Kaufmann W, Hossmann K-A,

Hossmann V (eds) Brain and heart infarct II. Springer, Berlin Heidelberg New York, pp 39–49

Zülch KJ (1981) Cerebrovascular pathology and pathogenesis as a basis of neuroradiological diagnosis. In: Diethelm L, Wende S (eds) Roentgendiagnosis of the central nervous system. Springer, Berlin Heidelberg New York, pp 1–192 (Handbuch der medizinischen Radiologie, vol XIV, part 1A)

Zülch KJ (1982) Correlated studies. In: Katsuki S, Tsubaki T, Toyokura Y (eds) Neurology. Proceedings of the 12th world congress of neurology, Kyoto, 1981. Excerpta Medica, Amsterdam

Zülch KJ (1983) Die Hirnleistungsinsuffizienz (HLI). Therapiewoche 33:1496–1511

Zülch KJ (1986) Brain Tumors. Their biology and pathology. 3rd edn. Springer, Berlin Heidelberg New York Tokyo (to be published)

Zülch KJ, Gessaga E (1972) Infarcts in the carotid system. Vasc Surg 6:114–119

Zülch KJ, Herberg HJ (1949) Das klinische Bild der akuten Blutsperre der Arteria carotis. Dtsch Z Nervenheilk 160:38–79

Zülch KJ, Kleihues P (1967) Neuropathology of cerebral infarction. In: Stroke. Thule international symposia 1966. Nordiska Bokhandelns, Stockholm, pp 57–75

Zülch KJ, Mennel HD, Zimmermann V (1974) Intracranial hypertension. In: Vinken PJ, Bruyn GW (eds) Tumors of the brain and skull. North-Holland, Amsterdam, pp 89–149 (Handbook of clinical neurology, vol 16, part I)

Name Index

Subject Index